HIV

MANUAL FOR
HEALTH CARE
PROFESSIONALS

H I V
MANUAL FOR
HEALTH CARE
PROFESSIONALS

Richard D. Muma, PA-C
Assistant Professor, Physician's Assistant Studies
School of Allied Health Sciences
Physician Assistant, Virology Research
Division of Infectious Diseases
Department of Internal Medicine
The University of Texas Medical Branch
Galveston, Texas

Barbara Ann Lyons, MA, PA-C
Associate Professor, Physician's Assistant Studies
School of Allied Health Sciences
Physician Assistant, Department of OB/GYN
The University of Texas Medical Branch
Galveston, Texas

Michael J. Borucki, MD
Assistant Professor, Virology Research
Division of Infectious Diseases
Department of Internal Medicine
The University of Texas Medical Branch
Galveston, Texas

Richard B. Pollard, MD
Professor, Microbiology and Internal Medicine
Chief, Virology Research
Division of Infectious Diseases
Department of Internal Medicine
The University of Texas Medical Branch
Galveston, Texas

APPLETON & LANGE
Norwalk, Connecticut

0-8385-0170-2

Notice: The authors and the publisher of this volume have taken care to make
certain that the doses of drugs and schedules of treatment are correct and
compatible with the standards generally accepted at the time of publication.
Nevertheless, as new information becomes available, changes in treatment
and in the use of drugs become necessary. The reader is advised to consult
the instruction and information material included in the package insert of
each drug or therapeutic agent before administration. This advice is
especially important when using new or infrequently used drugs. The
publisher disclaims any liability, loss, injury, or damage incurred as a
consequence, directly or indirectly, of the use or application of any of the
contents of this volume.

94 95 96 97 98 / 10 9 8 7 6 5 4 3 2 1

Prentice Hall International (UK) Limited, *London*
Prentice Hall of Australia Pty. Limited, *Sydney*
Prentice Hall Canada, Inc., *Toronto*
Prentice Hall Hispanoamericana, S.A., *Mexico*
Prentice Hall of India Private Limited, *New Delhi*
Prentice Hall of Japan, Inc., *Tokyo*
Simon & Schuster Asia Pte. Ltd., *Singapore*
Editora Prentice Hall do Brasil Ltda., *Rio de Janeiro*
Prentice Hall, *Englewood Cliffs, New Jersey*

Library of Congress Cataloging-in-Publication Data
HIV manual for health care professionals / Richard D. Muma . . . [et al.]
        p.   cm.
    Earlier version published with title: AIDS resource manual for physician
assistant students. 1992.
    Includes bibliographical references.
    ISBN 0-8385-0170-2
    1. HIV infections—Patients—Care—Handbooks, manuals, etc. I.
Muma, Richard D. II. Title: AIDS resource manual for physician assistant
students.
    [DNLM: 1. HIV infections—nursing. WD 308 H676457 1994]
RC607.A26H576 1994
616.97'92—dc20
DNLM/DLC
for Library of Congress   93-11164
                                                                                      CIP

Acquisitions Editor: Cheryl L. Mehalik
Production Editor: Sondra Greenfield
Production Services: Peter Strupp/Princeton Editorial Associates
Designer: Janice Barsevich Bielawa

PRINTED IN THE UNITED STATES OF AMERICA

CONTENTS

Contributors xiii

Preface xviii

Acknowledgments xx

1. **Introduction** 1

2. **Epidemiology** 7
   Statistics 7
   Origin, Transmission, and Transmission
      Groups 7
   Modes of Transmission 9
   Demographic Characteristics of AIDS in the
      United States 10
      Age 10
      Sex 11
      Race 11
   Geographic Distribution in the United States 11
   Disease Associated with AIDS 11
   CDC AIDS Definition for Adults 12

3. **Immunology** 15

4. **Etiology and Pathogenesis** 21

5. **Pre- and Posttest Counseling** 27

Pretest Counseling 29
Posttest Counseling 30
   Negative Test Result 30
   Positive Test Result 31

6. **Treatment of the Primary Infection and**
   Vaccines 35
   Treatment of the Primary Infection 35
   Vaccines 35

7. **Diagnosis and Treatment of Common**
   Infections and Malignancies 41
   Introduction 41
   HIV and Persistent Generalized
      Lymphadenopathy 42
     Clinical Manifestations 42
     Diagnosis 42
     Treatment 43
   Pneumocystis carinii Pneumonia 43
     Clinical Manifestations 44
     Diagnosis 47
     Treatment 47
   Histoplasmosis 49
     Clinical Manifestations 49
     Diagnosis 50
     Treatment 50
   Mycobacterium tuberculosis 51
     Clinical Manifestations 51
     Diagnosis 52
     Treatment 52
   Central Nervous System Toxoplasmosis . . 53
     Clinical Manifestations 53
     Diagnosis 54
     Treatment 54
   Cryptococcal Meningitis 55
     Clinical Manifestations 56

Diagnosis 56
Treatment 57
Primary Brain Lymphoma 58
Clinical Manifestations 58
Diagnosis 59
Treatment 60
AIDS Dementia Complex 60
Clinical Manifestations 61
Diagnosis 61
Treatment 61
Cytomegalovirus 62
Clinical Manifestations 64
Diagnosis 65
Treatment 65
Oral and Esophageal Candidiasis 66
Clinical Manifestations 66
Diagnosis 66
Treatment 66
Cryptosporidium 67
Clinical Manifestations 68
Diagnosis 68
Treatment 68
Mycobacterium avium Complex 69
Clinical Manifestations 69
Diagnosis 70
Treatment 70

8. Hepatitis 77
Introduction 77
Epidemiology 78
Clinical Manifestations 79
Acute Hepatitis 79
Chronic Hepatitis 79
Diagnosis 82
Management 82
Acute Hepatitis 82

| | Chronic Hepatitis | . . . . | 83 |
| | Summary | . . . . | 84 |

9.	**Syphilis**	87
	Clinical Manifestations	87
	Primary Syphilis	87
	Secondary Syphilis	89
	Latent Syphilis	89
	Tertiary Syphilis	90
	Neurosyphilis	90
	Diagnosis	91
	Treatment	95

10.	**Recognition and Management of Adverse**	
	Drug Reactions	99
	Introduction	99
	Definition	100
	Getting Started—Reviewing the Medication	
	Regimen	100
	Recognition	100
	Management	101
	Peripheral Neuropathy	104
	Comment	104
	Drugs	104
	Risk Factors for Drug-Induced Peripheral	
	Neuropathy	104
	Recognition	104
	Management	105
	Pancreatitis	105
	Comment	105
	Drugs	105
	Risk Factors for Drug-Induced Pancreatitis	106
	Recognition	106
	Management	106
	Renal Dysfunction	106
	Comment	106

Drugs 107

Risk Factors for Drug-Induced Renal
Dysfunction 107

Recognition 107

Management 107

Neutropenia 108

Comment 108

Drugs 108

Risk Factors 108

Recognition 108

Management 109

11. **Interpreting Laboratory Data** 111

Establishing the Diagnosis of HIV 112

Absolute T4 (CD4) Count 113

Abnormalities in Hematological Studies . . . 116

Abnormalities in Renal Function 119

Abnormalities in Liver Function 120

Abnormalities in Pancreatic Function 121

12. **Dermatologic Manifestations** 123

Infectious 124

Viral Infections 124

Fungal Infections 127

Noninfectious 129

Neoplastic 133

Kaposi's Sarcoma 133

13. **Women and HIV** 137

The Epidemiology of AIDS in Women 137

Diagnosis 138

HIV Testing in Women 138

Initial Work-up for Women with HIV 139

Medical Complications in Women with HIV
Infection 139

Human Papillomavirus and Cervical Disease 139

Herpes Simplex Virus	140
Chancroid	140
Syphilis	140
HIV Genital Ulcers	141
Pelvic Inflammatory Disease	141
Vaginal Candidiasis	142
Pregnancy	142
Management at Delivery and Postpartum .	144
Family Planning	145
Psychosocial Aspects of HIV in Women . .	146
Summary	146

14. Evaluation of Adult Patients Infected with HIV **149**
Evaluation of the Patient	152
History	152
Risk Factors	153
Medical History	153
Review of Systems	154
Physical Examination	159
Mouth	159
Eyes	159
Skin	160
Central and Peripheral Nervous System .	161
Lungs	162
Heart	163
Lymph Nodes	163
Abdomen	163
Genitalia and Rectum	164
Laboratory and Diagnostic Evaluation . . .	164
Asymptomatic and High Risk	165
Symptomatic HIV Infection or AIDS . . .	166
Psychosocial Evaluation and Patient Education	170

15. Pediatric HIV Infection **177**
| The Epidemiology of Pediatric AIDS . . . . | 177 |
| Diagnosis . . . . | 177 |

Laboratory Evaluation 178
HIV Testing in Children 180
Infectious Complications of HIV Infection in
  Children 182
  Pneumocystis carinii Pneumonia 182
  Lymphoid Interstitial Pneumonia 184
  Tuberculosis 184
  Respiratory Syncytial Virus 185
Congenital Syphilis and AIDS 186
Prophylaxis for PCP 195
Zidovudine Treatment for Children 196
Immunizations for HIV-Positive Children . . 197
Periodic Evaluation of Infants Born to
  HIV-Positive Mothers 197
Psychosocial Aspects of HIV in Children and
  Adolescents 197

16. **Social Worker Assessment and Intervention** 203
Evaluation of the Person Who Is HIV Positive
  or Has AIDS 204
Interventions 207
Community Resources 211

17. **Dentistry and AIDS** 213
Oral Candidiasis 215
Hairy Leukoplakia 215
Oral Recurrent Herpes Simplex 216
HIV Gingivitis, HIV Necrotizing Gingivitis,
  and HIV Periodontitis 216

18. **Nursing Assessment of HIV-Positive Patients** 217
Self-Assessment 218
Communication 219
Patient Assessment 221
  Anxiety 221
  Physical Assessment 223

Psychosocial Assessment 223
Grief Stages 224
Social Support 225

19. Outpatient Nursing 229
Outpatient Procedures 229
Indwelling Vascular Access Catheters . . . 234
Blood Transfusion 236
Lumbar Puncture/Bone Marrow Aspiration
  and Biopsy 241
Patient Education 242

20. Prevention 243
Modes of Transmission 243
Reducing Risk of HIV Transmission 244
  Individual Risk Reduction 244
  Health Care Worker Risk Reduction . . . 247
Prevention in Minority Populations 252
  Theories of the Epidemiology of HIV . . . 253
  Fear of Homosexuality/Bisexuality . . . 254
  Disbelief of Prevention Messages 255
  Poverty 256
  Differences in Language and Culture and
    Their Effect on Communication 257

21. Social and Psychological Aspects of AIDS . 261
Psychological Adaptation 261
Psychological Distress and Psychiatric
  Disorders 264
Response of Care Givers 266
Management Guidelines 268

Bibliography 271

Index 281

Contributors

Ayachi, Salah, PhD, PA-C
Associate Professor
Physician's Assistant Studies
School of Allied Health Sciences
Physician Assistant
Virology Research
Division of Infectious Diseases
Department of Internal Medicine
The University of Texas Medical Branch
Galveston, Texas

Borucki, Michael J., MD
Assistant Professor
Virology Research
Division of Infectious Diseases
Department of Internal Medicine
The University of Texas Medical Branch
Galveston, Texas

Bruhn, John G., PhD
Vice President for Academic Affairs and Research
The University of Texas at El Paso
El Paso, Texas

Carnes, Barbara A., RN, CS, PhD
Assistant Professor
Department of Mental Health/Management

School of Nursing
The University of Texas Medical Branch
Galveston, Texas

Curry, Janice G., PA-C
Physician Assistant
Virology Research
Division of Infectious Diseases
Department of Internal Medicine
The University of Texas Medical Branch
Galveston, Texas

Fuchs, John E., Jr., PharmD
Coordinator of Clinical Sciences
Department of Pharmaceutical Services
The University of Texas Medical Branch
Galveston, Texas

Hausrath, Stephen G., MD
Assistant Professor
Virology Research
Division of Infectious Diseases
Department of Internal Medicine
The University of Texas Medical Branch
Galveston, Texas

Lyon, T. C., Jr., DDS, PhD
Professor (Retired)
Department of Community Health and Preventive Dentistry
Baylor College of Dentistry, Dallas, Texas

Lyons, Barbara Ann, MA, PA-C
Associate Professor
Physician's Assistant Studies
School of Allied Health Sciences
Physician Assistant
Department of OB/GYN
The University of Texas Medical Branch
Galveston, Texas

Martens, Mark G., MD
Associate Professor
Department of OB/GYN
The University of Texas Medical Branch
Galveston, Texas

Montgomerie, Bernadette M., RN
Coordinator
Virology Research
Division of Infectious Diseases
Department of Internal Medicine
The University of Texas Medical Branch
Galveston, Texas

Muma, Richard D., PA-C
Assistant Professor
Physician's Assistant Studies
School of Allied Health Sciences
Physician Assistant
Virology Research
Division of Infectious Diseases
Department of Internal Medicine
The University of Texas Medical Branch
Galveston, Texas

Newman, Teresa A., PA-C
Assistant Professor
Physician's Assistant Studies
School of Allied Health Sciences
Physician Assistant
Department of OB/GYN
The University of Texas Medical Branch
Galveston, Texas

Ortega, Miguel A., MSW, ACSW, CSW-ACP
Supervisor
Department of Social Work

The University of Texas Medical Branch
Galveston, Texas

Paar, David P., MD
Assistant Professor
Virology Research
Division of Infectious Diseases
Department of Internal Medicine
The University of Texas Medical Branch
Galveston, Texas

Pollard, Richard B., MD
Professor
Microbiology and Internal Medicine
Chief, Virology Research
Division of Infectious Diseases
Department of Internal Medicine
The University of Texas Medical Branch
Galveston, Texas

Pounds, Janice, RN
Registered Nurse
AIDS Inpatient Unit
John Sealy Hospital
The University of Texas Medical Branch
Galveston, Texas

Roquemore, Sandee W., PA-C
Physician Assistant
Virology Research
Division of Infectious Diseases
Department of Internal Medicine
The University of Texas Medical Branch
Galveston, Texas

Stephenson, Karen S., PA-C
Assistant Professor
Physician's Assistant Studies
School of Allied Health Sciences

Physician Assistant
Department of Pediatrics
The University of Texas Medical Branch
Galveston, Texas

Wegmann, Angela, PA-C
Physician Assistant
Virology Research
Division of Infectious Diseases
Department of Internal Medicine
The University of Texas Medical Branch
Galveston, Texas

Contributing Author and Consultant

Valentine, Peggy, EdD, PA-C
Associate Professor
Physician Assistant Program
Director
National AIDS Minority Information and
  Education Program
Howard University
Washington, D.C.

....

....

....

PREFACE

The care of chronically ill patients with many complex problems can be difficult for a single clinician to manage. Often, many types of health care providers are needed to help manage the numerous medical and psychosocial concerns of the patient. Such is the care of HIV-positive patients; it is multifaceted and multidisciplinary.

HIV Manual for Health Care Professionals is intended for a variety of health care disciplines. When the book was piloted, we found it to be useful in training physicians, physician assistants, nurse practitioners, nurses, physical therapists, occupational therapists, psychologists, and social workers. Because the book describes a multidisciplinary approach to the care of HIV-positive patients, others not already mentioned may find the book to be useful as well.

A strength of this book is that it provides useful and practical information to the clinician on how to manage the HIV-positive and/or AIDS patient. A common comment from students and clinicians is that it is readable and provides current and concise information on all aspects of care.

All parts of the book provide a step-by-step approach to care, whether it be managing *Pneumocystis carinii* pneumonia, deciding on treatment for HIV, prevention counseling, or crisis intervention, as with suicide. The book is in a pocket guide format so that the student or clinician may refer to it whenever necessary.

The *HIV Manual* begins with a chapter on the multi-disciplinary approach to HIV patient care, and it is here where one can see how important a team approach is in managing HIV-positive patients. After the introductory material, the reader can review the current epidemiology, immunology, etiology, and pathogenesis of HIV, if necessary. A chapter on pretest and posttest counseling offers information on how to counsel individuals on HIV testing. This is followed by material on treatment of the primary infection, and information is given on current treatments such as zidovudine (AZT or ZDV), didanosine (ddI), and zalcitabine (ddC).

The next three chapters discuss in great detail the common diseases either directly or indirectly associated with HIV. It is here the reader will find the information needed to manage these diseases. The remaining text offers information on special issues frequently encountered in the care of HIV-positive patients, such as recognition and management of adverse drug reactions; interpreting laboratory data; dermatologic manifestations; and evaluation of adult, female, and pediatric patients, as well as social and psychological aspects of HIV and AIDS. Chapters are also included on social worker and nursing assessment, outpatient nursing, prevention, and dentistry and AIDS.

Each chapter is referenced with current reviews and studies on the corresponding topic, and there is an extensive bibliography at the end of the book for the individual who wishes to pursue any topic in greater detail.

The overall goal of this book is to provide the health care student or clinician with concise, up-to-date information on the HIV infection so that the care of HIV-infected patients can be optimized.

Richard D. Muma
Barbara Ann Lyons
Michael J. Borucki
Richard B. Pollard

ACKNOWLEDGMENTS

This book is dedicated to the HIV-positive patients and their health care providers at The University of Texas Medical Branch in Galveston, Texas.

We also acknowledge the input of our students who have helped shape the contents of this book, the cooperation of our contributing authors, and the continuing support of our faculty colleagues. We would like to thank our editor, Cheryl Mehalik of Appleton & Lange, for her interest in the book and her helpfulness throughout the production of the manuscript.

Preparation of this book was supported, in part, by the United States Department of Health and Human Services, Health Resources and Services Administration, Bureau of Health Professions, grant numbers 5D21 PE16001-11; 5D21 PE16001-12; 1U76 PE00238-01.

Chapter One

....

....

....

....

INTRODUCTION

RICHARD B. POLLARD, MD

On June 5, 1981, the *Morbidity and Mortality Weekly Report* (*MMWR*) carried an article reporting five cases of *Pneumocystis carinii* pneumonia (PCP) in homosexual men.[1] Within a short time, similar cases had been reported in New York and San Francisco, while other reports included cases of perianal herpes and uncontrollable diarrhea, all unresponsive to treatment and occurring in homosexual men.

Additionally, other rare opportunistic infections such as *Mycobacterium avium-intracellulare* were reported increasingly in adults, and several patients were infected with *Cryptosporidium,* a disease so rare that only a few cases were known to have occurred in prior years. Reports of non-Hodgkin's lymphoma and Kaposi's sarcoma (KS) in homosexual men further complicated the puzzling medical picture. These occurrences marked the emergence of what appeared to be a new disease, known as Acquired Immunodeficiency Syndrome (AIDS).

Since the recognition of AIDS and its causative agent, human immunodeficiency virus (HIV), more than 200,000 cases have been diagnosed in the United States.[2] Many more are expected to be diagnosed within the next two years as the Centers for Disease Control and Prevention (CDC) implements its new AIDS case definition.[3]

As with any disease, trends of its occurrence in populations tend to change over time, AIDS is no different. In 1981, 189 cases of AIDS were reported to the CDC from 15 states and the District of Columbia; 76% of cases were reported from New York and California.[4] Ninety-seven percent of cases reported were among men, 79% of whom reported being homosexual/bisexual; no cases were reported among children.[4] In 1990, more than 43,000 cases were reported from all states, the District of Columbia, and U.S. territories; more than 11% of adolescent and adult cases were in women; and nearly 800 cases were in children.[4] The CDC expects between 47,000 and 85,000 new cases in 1993 and between 43,000 and 93,000 new cases in 1994.[5] Through 1994, a cumulative total between 415,000 and 535,000 is expected.[5]

It should be mentioned that most of the patients currently seeking HIV care were infected before the discovery of the virus and before significant public health measures were developed. Hence, predicting the future course of the infection is hampered by the lack of data concerning new HIV infections that are now occurring and will only present for medical attention in the latter half of this decade. Therefore, these individuals will not be represented in the demographic statistics until they seek medical care. This lag period makes the development of public health strategies for this particular situation much more complicated than for other infectious agents.

The other major influence of the changing epidemiology has been a shift in the burden of HIV care, which has occurred since the epidemic began. While many of the early patients, who were injecting drug users and indigent, requiring the use of public hospital facilities, a large number of the initially infected male homosexuals were employed and had health care insurance. This is a significantly different population from that projected in the figure. The patients newly acquiring HIV infection, because of socioeconomic status and racial and other demographic factors, are expected to primarily utilize public health facilities as their major resource for health care. This will further increase the influence of the epidemic on large public hospitals, university referral centers, and, in an overall sense, involve a patient group that has limited access to adequate health care.

Another major shift in HIV care has been the rapid development of therapies for the primary infection as well as for many opportunistic infections. The development of therapies in this particular arena has been both dramatic and rapid. While no single therapeutic advance has altered the course of the epidemic, new single agents and more recently combination agent therapy directed at HIV, as well as the development of preventative therapy for many of the opportunistic infections, have dramatically affected the outcomes of many patients with HIV infection.

Almost every group of health care providers has been involved in the care of HIV-infected patients to date. The physician groups most affected, and involved early, included adult and pediatric infectious disease specialists and oncologists. These two groups continue to be very active in AIDS care and research. In addition, a large group of primary care physicians, including general internists and family practitioners, has increasingly provided health care for this ever-increasing group of patients.

Physician extenders have also been impacted by the HIV epidemic. Nurse practitioners and physician assistants have been heavily involved in the care of patients with HIV infection. Such individuals have been particularly useful and skillful in providing primarily outpatient care. Both groups have been involved in clinical research projects and have proven to be an excellent resource.

The impact of the nursing profession has also been significant. Many institutions have developed specialized nursing units, inpatient and outpatient, and nurses have been required to develop significant knowledge concerning the care of HIV-infected individuals. In addition, nurses have also served as a major resource for clinical research and have contributed greatly to the development of new knowledge.

Another group that has been impacted are social workers. They have participated heavily in the development of resources for HIV-infected patients. Social workers have played a major role in the identification of public assistance programs and the enabling of patients to become users of medicare, medicaid, housing, free medication programs, and the like. Many institutions have developed specialized social workers who deal primarily with HIV-infected patients.

Additional groups of health care providers, such as occupational therapists and physical therapists, have also participated in the care of HIV-infected individuals, particularly those patients who have prolonged hospital stays that require rehabilitation in order to maximize their ability to function. Dietitians provide consultation and prescribe dietary regimens for those individuals who need to gain weight or require parenteral nutrition. Hospital-based clergy, ethicists, and other individuals in the medical humanities have also participated in the development of policies for the provision of care for large numbers of HIV-infected individuals. This latter group has provided comfort to individual patients as well as assistance in developing appropriate policies for health care providers.

While it is difficult to predict the future in any medical area, it would seem obvious that this epidemic will be marked considerably by therapeutic advances. These will no doubt occur in a progressive fashion, with the development of a universally effective solution to HIV infection probably not forthcoming in the near future. More likely, there will be the continued development of combinations of therapeutic agents directed at the primary infection, along with the development of multiple therapies for opportunistic infections and continued emphasis on the development of prophylactic agents for opportunistic infections.

It is expected that the patients identified earlier in their HIV infection will have an increasingly improved prognosis and a prolonged life span. Their quality of life will also begin to be affected significantly with fewer hospitalizations and a much greater emphasis on outpatient therapy. The necessity for detection of HIV-infected individuals as these therapies become widespread will require aggressive attempts to identify infected patients much earlier than at present. As the patient numbers increase, a significant amount of attention to the development of medication resources will be required. Newer therapies, which will be expensive and yet prolong life, will require consideration for their adequate provision. In general, there should be optimism that this infection will be impacted by therapeutic advances and increases in knowledge about HIV itself and the immunologic perturbations associated with infection. This may translate into a chronic manageable disease with a significantly prolonged life span for each HIV-infected individual. One is cautiously optimistic that dramatic but gradually progressive changes will occur until this epidemic is controlled by changes in medical therapy over the foreseeable future.

The following text, which will attempt to bring together fundamental information regarding HIV and AIDS, is intended as a guide to assist the clinician in understanding the epidemiology, etiology, clinical manifestations, treatment, and management of HIV and AIDS. Since the data regarding HIV and AIDS are changing almost daily as new information is uncovered, future research could reveal information that is contrary to that presented in this text or that alters the significance of particular facts or theories. To the best of our knowledge, the information that follows is accurate at the time of this printing.

References

1. Centers for Disease Control. *Pneumocystis* pneumonia—Los Angeles. *MMWR.* 1981;30:250–252.
2. Centers for Disease Control. Statistics. *AIDS.* 1993;7: 145–147.
3. Centers for Disease Control and Prevention. 1993 revised classification system for HIV infection and expanded surveillance case definition for AIDS among adolescents and adults. *MMWR.* 1992;41(RR-17):1–19.
4. Centers for Disease Control. Update: acquired immunodeficiency syndrome—United States, 1982–1990. *MMWR.* 1991;40:358–369.
5. Centers for Disease Control and Prevention. Projections of the number of persons diagnosed with AIDS and the number of immunosuppressed HIV-infected persons—United States, 1992–1994. *MMWR.* 1992;41 (RR-18):1–29.

Chapter Two

....

....

....

....

EPIDEMIOLOGY

RICHARD D. MUMA, PA-C
MICHAEL J. BORUCKI, MD

■ Statistics

As mentioned in the previous chapter, the number of AIDS cases has increased rapidly. Between June 5, 1981 and December 31, 1992, 253,448 AIDS cases (adult/adolescent subtotal = 249,199; pediatric subtotal = 4,249) were reported in the United States.[1] More than 600,000 have been reported worldwide.[2] The number is expected to grow considerably over the next several years. The World Health Organization estimates that 8 to 10 million adults and 1 million children worldwide are infected with HIV. By the year 2000, 40 million persons may be infected with HIV.[3]

■ Origin, Transmission, and Transmission Groups

Manifestations of AIDS were noted as early as 1979 after various reports from Africa, Haiti, and the United States

TABLE 2–1. ADULT AIDS CASES BY TRANSMISSION GROUPS. UNITED STATES (MALE AND FEMALE) THROUGH DECEMBER 1992[1]

Transmission Groups	No.	%
Men who have sex with men	142,626	57
Injecting drug use	57,412	23
Men who have sex with men and inject drugs	15,899	6
Hemophilia/coagulation disorder	2,026	1
Heterosexual contact	16,254	7
Recipient of blood transfusions, blood components, or tissue	4,980	2
Undetermined	10,002	4
TOTAL	249,199	100

documented rare opportunistic infections and neoplasms in supposedly healthy individuals. Epidemiologic evidence *suggests* that the virus may have first appeared in Africa.[4] However, many different theories have been hypothesized to explain the origin of the disease. Viruses that strongly resemble HIV endemically infect African green monkeys without causing disease in them. It is postulated that a mutation in one of these viruses resulted in HIV and was transmitted to man, most likely by trauma.

AIDS cases in adults and adolescents have occurred in six major transmission groups.[1] These groups are arranged in a hierarchy so that patients with multiple risks are placed in only one group. The distribution of AIDS patients by groups in the United States is outlined in Table 2–1. The majority of U.S. AIDS cases occur in homosexual and bisexual men. This is beginning to change as more cases are reported in injecting drug users (IDUs) and heterosexual males and females.[5] Because the interval from infection until symptoms is estimated to be

11+ years, these changes in HIV transmission patterns will not be reflected in the AIDS statistics for another decade. In Africa and Haiti, the number of reported AIDS cases is highest among heterosexuals. Heterosexual contact is the presumed mode of transmission within those countries.[5]

■ Modes of Transmission

HIV is transmitted in limited ways: through sexual contact, through infected blood components and clotting factor concentrates, and perinatally. HIV has been isolated from a number of body fluids, including blood, saliva, semen, urine, cerebrospinal fluid, and sweat. The virus preferentially infects helper T (also known as T4+, CD4+, OKT4+) lymphocytes and conceivably could be recovered from any site where such cells are found. However, such findings are not necessarily significant in the context of public health. There is no evidence that contact with saliva or tears results in infection with HIV.

Actions and/or behaviors that are considered high risk and are frequently associated with HIV infection include vaginal and/or receptive anal intercourse and other potentially traumatic sexual activities with HIV-infected individuals. Examples are included below.

- Anilingus: Encircling the anal area with the tongue.
- Cunnilingus: Tonguing the vagina/clitoris (more risky during menstrual period).
- Fellatio: Tonguing and sucking the male genital area (more risky if partner ejaculates in the mouth).
- Fisting: Putting hand, fist, or forearm into the rectum or vagina.
- Urolagnia: Urinating on the skin (more risky if there are open cuts in the skin, mouth, vagina, or rectum).

- Rectal and/or vaginal placement of objects: Placing objects (ie, sex toys) may cause tears in the mucosa, which could serve as a portal of entry for the virus.
- Needle sharing and frequent injection of IV drugs.
- Hemophiliacs, and others, necessitating blood transfusions prior to mid-1985. Blood components that presumably have transmitted HIV include whole blood, red cells, platelets, and plasma.
- Maternal–fetal transmission: HIV-infected women transmit HIV to the fetus or infant either in utero or at delivery in 25% to 35% of cases.[6]

Actions and/or behaviors that are considered low risk and usually not associated with HIV infection include:

- Occupational transmission: The collective evidence strongly suggests that the risk to health care workers of occupational transmission (needle sticks) of HIV is low (less than 0.4% or 1:200)[7] and can be most effectively reduced by following recommended guidelines for the care of HIV-infected persons and the handling of their specimens (see Chapter 20).
- Casual contact: There is no evidence that AIDS or HIV can be transmitted through air, food, water, fomites, arthropods (mosquitos), or by casual contact (ie, hugging or kissing).

■ Demographic Characteristics of AIDS in the United States

Age
Eighty-eight percent of all AIDS patients reported to the CDC are between the ages of 20 and 49.[5]

Sex

Approximately 90% of adult and adolescent AIDS patients are men.[1] Of these men with AIDS, 64% are homosexual/bisexual, and another 20% are heterosexual IDUs.[1] Men in other transmission groups account for 15% of the total cases. Half of the women are IDUs, and more than 34% have histories of sexual contact with men at high risk for AIDS or who were born in countries where heterosexual contact is believed to be the major mode of transmission.[1] Approximately 7% of women with AIDS are blood transfusion recipients. The remaining 9% are undetermined.[1]

Race

In adults and adolescents, 53% of AIDS cases occur in whites, 29% in African-Americans, 17% in Hispanics, and 0.8% in Asian/Pacific Islander and American Indian/Alaskan natives. In children, 21% of AIDS occurs in whites, 54% in African-Americans, 24% in Hispanics, and 0.7% in Asian/Pacific Islander and American Indican/Alaskan natives.[1]

■ Geographic Distribution in the United States

All 50 states, the District of Columbia, and the U.S. territories have reported at least one AIDS case. Two states, California and New York, account for 72.9 cases per 100,000 population reported through September 1992.[8] Florida accounted for 37.1 cases per 100,000 population, Texas, 16.9, and New Jersey, 26.4.[8]

■ Disease Associated with AIDS

The two most commonly reported diseases seen in adult patients with AIDS are *Pneumocystis carinii* pneumonia and Kaposi's sarcoma.[1] Other opportunistic illnesses associated with AIDS are seen less frequently. Of these, esophageal candidiasis is the most common.[1] Less commonly reported infections include cytomegalovirus infection, cryptococcus, atypical mycobacteriosis, chronic herpes simplex, cryptosporidiosis, and toxoplasmosis.[1] However, with longer survival rates, less common illnesses are likely to occur more often.

■ CDC AIDS Definition for Adults

In the mid-1980s the CDC developed a surveillance case definition for AIDS in adults and adolescents (aged 13 and over), and children (less than 13 years of age) in order to track the disease. The definition for children is discussed in Chapter 15. The adult and adolescent definition was based on the early observation that patients with AIDS developed certain opportunistic illnesses secondary to a specific defect in a cell-mediated component of the immune system. If no other cause for the cellular immune dysfunction was present, the diagnosis of one of 12 opportunistic illnesses was considered indicative of AIDS. In 1987 the CDC revised this definition (Table 2–2) to include HIV dementia, HIV wasting syndrome, and other illnesses.[9] More recently the CDC has expanded the AIDS surveillance definition to include all HIV-infected persons who have fewer than 200 T4 cells/mm^3, or a T4 cell percentage of total lymphocytes of less than 14.[10] This expansion also includes three conditions—pulmonary tuberculosis, recurrent pneumonia, and invasive cervical cancer—and retains the 23 conditions in the case definition published in 1987.[9,10] Refer to Chapter 14 for the new CDC classification system and how it reflects the new AIDS case definition.

TABLE 2–2. LIST OF CONDITIONS IN THE 1987 AIDS ADULT AND ADOLESCENT SURVEILLANCE CASE DEFINITION[9]

- Candidiasis of bronchi, trachea, or lungs
- Candidiasis, esophageal
- Coccidioidomycosis, disseminated or extrapulmonary
- Cryptococcoses, extrapulmonary
- Cryptosporidiosis, chronic intestinal (>1 month duration)
- Cytomegalovirus disease (other than liver, spleen, or nodes)
- Cytomegalovirus retinitis (with loss of vision)
- HIV encephalopathy
- Herpes simplex: chronic ulcer(s) (>1 month duration); or bronchitis, pneumonitis, or esophagitis
- Histoplasmosis, disseminated or extrapulmonary
- Isosporiasis, chronic intestinal (>1 month duration)
- Kaposi's sarcoma
- Lymphoma, Burkitt's (or equivalent term)
- Lymphoma, immunoblastic (or equivalent term)
- Lymphoma, primary in brain
- *Mycobacterium avium* complex or *M. kansasii,* disseminated or extrapulmonary
- *Mycobacterium tuberculosis,* disseminated or extrapulmonary
- *Mycobacterium,* other species or unidentified species, disseminated or extrapulmonary
- *Pneumocystis carinii* pneumonia
- Progressive multifocal leukoencephalopathy
- *Salmonella* septicemia, recurrent
- Toxoplasmosis of brain
- Wasting syndrome caused by HIV

References

1. Centers for Disease Control and Prevention. *HIV/AIDS Surveillance Report,* February 1993:1–23.
2. Statistics from the World Health Organization. *AIDS.* 1993;7:297–298.
3. World Health Organization. In point of fact. Geneva: World Health Organization, May 1991 (no.74).

4. Anderson RM, May RM. Understanding the AIDS pandemic. *Sci Am.* 1992;5:58–66.

5. Centers for Disease Control. Update: acquired immunodeficiency syndrome—United States. *MMWR.* 1991;40:358–369.

6. Nanda D. Human immunodeficiency virus infection in pregnancy. *Obstet Gynecol Clin North Am.* 1990;17: 617–626.

7. Centers for Disease Control. Recommendations for preventing transmission of human immunodeficiency virus and hepatitis B virus to patients during exposure-prone invasive procedures. *MMWR.* 1991; 40(RR-8):1–9.

8. Centers for Disease Control. Quarterly AIDS map. *MMWR.* 1992;41:805.

9. Centers for Disease Control. Revision of the CDC surveillance case definition for acquired immunodeficiency syndrome. *MMWR.* 1987;36:1s–15s.

10. Centers for Disease Control and Prevention. 1993 revised classification system for HIV infection and expanded surveillance case definition for AIDS among adolescents and adults. *MMWR.* 1992;41(RR-17):1–19.

Chapter Three

IMMUNOLOGY

MICHAEL J. BORUCKI, MD

Immunity is a normal adaptive response. It protects the body from invasion by microbial agents and prevents proliferation of mutant cells, such as those involved in neoplastic growth.

Most of our knowledge of the immune system has arisen through "natural experiments" in which persons have defects in immunity as a consequence of inherited or congenital defects, for example, severe combined immunodeficiency (SCID) syndrome in children. Through such "natural experiments," it was recognized that the normal immune response develops in two parallel arms: one humoral ("humor" referring to one of the various bodily fluids, hence soluble) and the other cellular. The descriptions, humoral and cellular, refer to the nature of the *effector* arm of the response; the humoral immune response is effected through antibodies, and the cellular immune response is effected through cells, largely cytotoxic T cells.

Both arms are initially dependent upon cells for recognition, processing, and presentation of foreign antigens.

Such antigen-presenting-cells (APCs) are usually of monocyte/macrophage origin and are unique in that they can recognize and react to a variety of foreign antigens without having previously been exposed to them. The APCs are unique in that they can respond to a wide diversity of foreign antigens. The APCs phagocytose the foreign antigen (bacteria, virus, parasites, tumor cells, transplanted tissue), process the antigen, and then display (present) the antigens on their surface so that other cells of the immune response (B and T cells) can recognize these antigens as foreign. As they mature, the B and T cells become "committed" to the specific antigen and once mature are primed to specifically recognize and target this one antigen. They may also respond to very closely related antigens but will not respond to antigens that are much different from their principal target antigen. The ability of the body's immune response to recognize the vast diversity of antigens then depends on the above scenario being repeated again and again as the body recognizes each new foreign antigen. In total, it is believed humans have the capacity to recognize perhaps 100 million distinct foreign antigens.

Once stimulated by the interaction of APC, foreign antigen, and various immune modulators (interferons and interleukins), B cells transform and divide in the process of clonal expansion. As the maturation process continues, the B cells become plasma cells that bear specific immunoglobulin (antibody, abbreviated Ig or Ab) on their surface and secrete immunoglobulins into the surrounding environment when stimulated. Plasma cells may remain dormant following the initial response until their surface immunoglobulins (sIg) encounter the specific antigens that began the cascade. The plasma cells' surface immunoglobulins and the secreted immunoglobulins react with the identical antigen.

In all, five classes of Ab are known: IgG, IgM, IgA, IgD, and IgE. The majority of circulating immunoglobulin in the bloodstream is of the IgG class in its four subclasses: IgG1, IgG2, IgG3, and IgG4. IgA (also called "secretory-Ab") is the dominant class in saliva, bronchial, and other mucous secretions. Following the first exposure to an antigen, immunoglobulins of the IgM class typically appear first and then are rapidly followed by a secondary homologous response with IgG-class antibody. The IgM class is a short-lived species that typically persists for approximately 6 months; the IgG class persists longer, usually for many years. This pattern of IgM appearance first, followed by IgG, is often used as a diagnostic aid since the IgM response is typically seen early and temporarily following an acute infection. IgD is the major surface immunoglobulin (sIg) on B cells, and IgE is the effector immunoglobulin of immediate (type I, allergic, anaphylaxis) hypersensitivity.

The cellular arm of the immune response is somewhat more complex and involves T cells of three distinct populations with different functions: helper, suppressor, and cytotoxic. The helper and suppressor functions serve to modulate the voracity of the cell-mediated effector response.

The helper cells promote or amplify the aggressiveness of the cell-mediated immune (CMI) response. T cells are often categorized by the markers they bear on their surfaces. For example, all mature T cells have a pan-T-cell marker on their surface called CD2 (also known as T3 or OKT3). Subpopulations of T cells may display other markers such as CD8 (T8 or OKT8) or CD4 (T4 or OKT4). These surface markers may suggest differing functions of these subpopulations of T cells; for example, most T cells with "helper" activity are phenotypically CD4 cells. CD4 cells thus represent a critical subpopulation of the cell-mediated arm of the immune response.

Human immunodeficiency virus binds to CD4 (OKT4) on the surface of CD4+ (helper) cells and thereafter enters and infects the cell. Over time, the helper/CD4+

population is progressively infected by HIV, and the critical helper functions are slowly lost. HIV also infects monocytes/macrophages, the antigen-presenting cells, and further compromises the ability of the immune system to react to new antigens (neoantigens) by impairing both the APC and the CD4 cells, which are critical to neoantigen responses.

CD4+ cells may also be suppressed without evidence of HIV infection, infection by related viruses, or other defined causes. This condition is referred to as idiopathic CD4+ T lymphocytopenia, or ICL.[1] ICL is heterogeneous in that it affects a demographically diverse population and has different clinical manifestations, both of which make it dissimilar from HIV infection and AIDS.[1] Further research is in progress to determine the significance of ICL and its relationship to HIV infection.

In addition, the CMI arm is responsible for controlling a variety of infections, among them *Pneumocystis carinii, Toxoplasma gondii,* cytomegalovirus, herpes virus, zoster virus, cryptosporidia, *Cryptococcus neoformans,* tuberculosis and related mycobacterioses, *Candida, Histoplasma,* and other mycoses. This group of infections commonly causes disease in patients with severely compromised cell-mediated immunity, like that seen in AIDS patients. It was the presence of these disorders occurring in previously well adults that alerted the medical community to a new syndrome of immune deficiency acquired after birth (not genetic/inherited).

In addition to its protective effects, cell-mediated immunity is responsible for delayed hypersensitivity, commonly defined as the sensitization of T cells to react with skin antigens. This is also referred to as a type IV cell-mediated response. An example would be transplant rejection.

It is clear how important both humoral and cell-mediated immunity are to one's body. If there is a de-

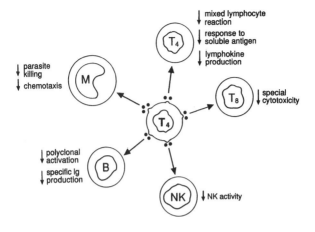

Figure 3–1. Consequences of a low T4 (CD4) blood cell count.

crease in CD4 helper cells, the following defects are often seen (Fig. 3–1):

- Decreased lymphocyte reaction
- Decreased response to soluble antigen (as demonstrated by anergy in skin testing)
- Decreased lymphokine production
- Decreased specific cytotoxicity
- Decreased killer cell activity
- Decreased polyclonal activation
- Decreased Ig production
- Decreased parasite killing
- Decreased chemotaxis

In summary, HIV infects CD4 cells (one of the orchestrators of the immune system). This, in turn, creates a major defect in the immune system, thereby causing the body to become susceptible to opportunistic infections and malignancies. Further research is under way, and other cells within the immune system have been found to be susceptible to infection with HIV. The exact consequence of the infection of other cell types is not clear.

Reference

1. CD4 positive T cell suppression among people without HIV clarified. *NIAID AIDS Agenda.* Winter 1993: 3–4.

Chapter Four

....
....
....
....

ETIOLOGY AND PATHOGENESIS

MICHAEL J. BORUCKI, MD

The human immunodeficiency virus is implicated as the causative agent in AIDS. This virus is a member of the family of viruses named retroviridae. The retroviruses have stimulated scientific interest for the past three decades, and much of the research has linked them to cancer and immune defects.

Retroviridae, or retroviruses, are so named for their unique ability to replicate in reverse fashion. These viruses have the ability to transfer their genetic information from RNA to DNA using an enzyme named reverse transcriptase (Fig. 4–1), which is the reverse of the usual processes of transcription (DNA to RNA) and translation (RNA to protein). Retroviruses are widespread among vertebrates and have been isolated from fish, reptiles, birds, and mammals. Among mammals and birds, virtually all species that have been examined closely have yielded retroviruses. Although retroviruses were initially identified with malignancies, it is apparent that they are

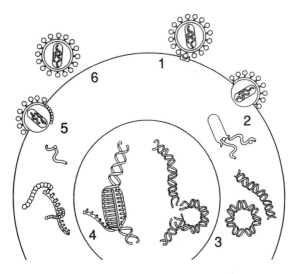

Figure 4–1. Life cycle of retroviruses. 1 = Binding of viruses to target cell. 2 = Uncoating of virus and transcription of viral RNA to DNA by reverse transcriptase. 3 = Viral DNA circularization and integration into host genome. 4 = Transcription and protein synthesis. 5 = Assembly of viral proteins and RNA at cell surface. 6 = Budding of mature viral particle from host.

associated with a wide variety of degenerative diseases, such as AIDS. Retroviruses are broadly divided into two classes: transforming retroviruses (oncogenic) and nontransforming (lentiviruses).

Compared to many other viruses, retroviruses are transmitted inefficiently from one host to another. This low transmission rate no doubt reflects the extreme lability of the virion. All retroviruses are readily inactivated by mild detergent, gentle heating, drying, or moderately high or low pH. Thus, transmission is unlikely except through close physical contact involving exchange of blood or other bodily fluids (as during sexual intercourse), or from mother to fetus. Most retrovirus infections, including HIV, are characterized by latency periods measured in months to years. Such long latency periods are clearly what one should expect for a virus whose major modes of transmission are either vertical or via intimate contact, since a virus that killed its host before it could be transmitted would not survive for very long in nature.

However, current studies indicate that, during the latency period, when there is little HIV replication in the blood, high levels of virus replication are found in the lymphoid tissue,[1] including the lymph nodes, spleen, tonsils, and adenoids. This information may prompt a rethinking of the optimal time to initiate treatment of HIV-infected patients.[2]

To continue, early epidemiologic evidence from patients with AIDS suggested a transmissible agent, probably a virus, particularly since the routes of transmission appeared to parallel those of hepatitis B virus: sexual contacts and exchange of blood or blood products. The slow and selective loss of the CD4 T-cell phenotype also suggested a particular affinity (tropism) for this cell type. Armed with this epidemiologic information and knowledge of how other infections are spread, the search began for the presumed etiologic agent of AIDS.

Because members of the human retroviridae were known to be T-cell leukemogenic and spread by close (principally sexual) contacts and/or blood products, much interest was devoted to searching for a new retrovirus as the putative agent for AIDS. Almost simultaneously, two groups—one French, headed by Luc Montagnier, and the other American, under the direction of Robert C. Gallo—isolated a retrovirus from patients with AIDS. The French group named the virus lymphadenopathy associated virus

(LAV); Gallo named it HTLV-III after the nomenclature of the previously identified T-cell leukemogenic retroviruses, HTLV-I and HTLV-II. The two viruses were subsequently shown to be the identical agent and by convention are now referred to as the human immunodeficiency virus-1 (HIV-1 or simply, HIV). A second human immunodeficiency virus has been isolated that causes a similar spectrum of disease, and it has been called HIV-2. Cases of HIV-2 in the United States have been reported only rarely.

The genome of HIV bears a strong resemblance to other retrovidridae and is principally organized into three coding segments: the group associated antigen protein components (GAG), the envelope (ENV), and the polymerase (POL) segments. HIV has additional sequences that code for regulatory components, including both positive (enhancing) and negative (inhibitory) functions.

The HIV-ENV gene codes for a 160-kilodalton (kD) protein that is cleaved into 120-kD (external) and 41-kD (transmembranous) portions. Both are glycosylated; glycoprotein 120 (gp120) binds to CD4 and is important in viral attachment to its target cells; glycoprotein 41 (gp41) is probably involved in infected cell–uninfected cell attachment and syncytium formation. Antibodies against both of these glycoproteins (or ENV components) are typically found in the blood of infected persons.

The GAG proteins are the principal structural components of the virus. One of them, a 24-kD protein, p24, may be found in the serum of infected persons and when present suggests active infection and virus growth. Some data suggest that the presence of antigen in the serum connotes a poorer prognosis. Patients infected with HIV will typically have circulating antibodies against one or more of the GAG proteins. It is the presence of these antibodies against GAG and ENV components that is tested in the screening (ELISA) blood test.

The POL gene codes for three principal components: the reverse transcriptase (RT), protease (PR), and integrase (IN). Reverse transcriptase is so called because rather than DNA being transcribed to RNA (the typical scenario), viral RNA is turned into DNA, hence "reverse" transcription. Since cells of the human host do not use such a process, the unique process of reverse transcription provides a useful avenue for therapy. Zidovudine (ZDV, or AZT), for example, acts through inhibition of reverse transcription. The protease cleaves the POL gene product into its three components. Although mammalian cells do use proteases to perform many cellular functions, the actions of these proteases tend to be very selective/specific, and thus inhibition of the HIV serine protease may provide another avenue for therapy. Indeed, clinical trials of protease inhibitors are in progress.

Since infection with HIV is a lifetime infection, extreme measures should be taken to prevent its further spread. One must remember that not everyone experiences symptoms once infected, and transmission can still occur when one is asymptomatic. Individuals at risk for acquiring HIV and those who have documented sexually transmitted diseases other than HIV should have counseling regarding HIV testing (refer to Chapter 5). If an individual agrees to testing, posttest counseling is recommended regardless of the results. Seronegative patients must be counseled that testing does not substitute for the prevention of risk behavior likely to result in the transmission of HIV; continued high-risk behavior poses a hazard regardless of testing.

References

1. Pantaleo G, Graziosi C, Demarest JF, et al. HIV infection is active and progressive in lymphoid tissue during the clinically latent stage of disease. *Nature.* 1993;362:355–358.

2. National Institute of Allergy and Infectious Diseases. National Institute of Health. HIV disease is active and progressive in lymphoid organs during clinical latency. *News from NIAID.* March 24, 1993:1–4.

Chapter Five

PRE- AND POSTTEST COUNSELING

TERESA A. NEWMAN, PA-C

During the initial encounter with a potential HIV-positive individual, a health professional must attempt to meet several specific goals. The encounter should not only be a "testing" session, but should also include discussion and counseling both before and after testing. There are important reasons for counseling with the HIV test. Counseling and testing affect the behavior of those at risk of becoming infected.[1] Their behavior should change to prevent infecting themselves or transmitting the disease to others. Counseling and testing help infected individuals to access medical care prior to progression to AIDS.

Prior to HIV counseling, the clinician should take a thorough drug and sexual history.[2] This assessment allows the clinician to ascertain what risks the individual may have for HIV. These questions may be difficult for the clinician to ask as well as for the individual to answer. It is best to start with open-ended questions and continue with specific, nonjudgmental questions. For instance, instead

TABLE 5–1. INDIVIDUALS AT RISK FOR HIV[3]

Children of HIV-infected mothers

Individuals from countries with a high rate of HIV-infected heterosexuals

Individuals with multiple sexual partners (eg, prostitutes)

Hemophiliacs

Homosexuals/bisexuals

Injecting drug users

Transfusion recipients, especially between 1978 and 1985

Sexual partners of HIV-infected persons, injecting drug users, or bisexuals

of asking individuals if they are "gay" or homosexual, ask if they have sex with men, women, or both.[2,3] The clinician should ask about the number of sexual partners and whether each partner injects drugs, is promiscuous, is at risk for HIV, or is bisexual.[3] When individuals may be unsure concerning these behaviors in their partners, testing should probably proceed, as not all partners would willingly disclose this information to their sexual partners. When asking about drug use, it may be easier to start with prescription drugs and work toward asking about IV and illicit drug use. Concurrently with drug/sexual partner questioning, the clinician can include education about how drugs and alcohol interfere with judgment and may promote unsafe sexual practices. If the individual is at risk for HIV (Table 5–1), then proceed with the HIV counseling and testing. If the individual does not have high-risk behavior or exposure, use the opportunity to educate the individual about HIV and AIDS.[2]

Additionally, the CDC recommends that acute-care facilities encourage health-care providers to ask every individual routinely about his or her HIV risks and to offer HIV counseling.[4] Furthermore, hospitals with an HIV seroprevalence rate of at least 1% or an AIDS diagnosis rate of ≥1.0 per 1000 discharges should strongly consider adopting a policy of offering HIV counseling and testing routinely to individuals ages 15 to 54.[4] In 1990, it was estimated that 10.6% of U.S. hospitals had an AIDS diagnosis rate of >1%.[5]

■ Pretest Counseling

When discussing HIV testing, the clinician should counsel the individual on the advantages and disadvantages of being tested as well as the limits of the test (see Chapter 11). The individual should also be asked to give informed consent prior to testing.[2] Advantages of being tested include receiving medical care early if the test result is positive, before AIDS develops.[3] It is also a time to encourage safe sexual practices that will decrease the individual's risk of being infected and/or decrease the risk of transmission to others. Discussion of intravenous drug use and needle sharing can be initiated. Written material on safe sexual practices and IV drug use are helpful for individuals to take with them but should not be used in place of counseling. Pretest counseling may relieve anxiety in those who are unlikely to be infected and may assist women with risk factors if they are planning a pregnancy.

If the individual requests testing, explore his or her reasons for wanting to be tested.[2] The psychological trauma of testing positive is one of the major disadvantages to testing (see Chapters 16 and 21). To help prepare the individual, the clinician should ask why the individual wants to be tested.[3] This is also the time to assess risk factors, to determine how likely the individual is to be positive, how the individual is expected to respond to the results, and what the individual will do with the information.

Pretest counseling is the time at which to discuss preventive measures the individual can develop.[2] Discussion of safe sexual practices, discontinuing intravenous drug use, and the effects of drugs and alcohol on judgment of safe sex should be done at this time. The individual should be counseled on the testing procedure and what the results of the HIV test could mean.[2,3] If the individual has had a recent exposure to HIV (within the past 6 weeks) the test result may be negative. The individual should be counseled to be retested in 3 to 6 months. Individuals should be warned about false-negative tests if they have been exposed to HIV more than 6 weeks earlier.

Before ending the counseling session, a follow-up appointment should be made to review test results and for posttest counseling.[2] This is a good time for individuals to review what they have learned and what methods of protection should be used in the future.

The consent form for HIV testing should include the purpose of the test and what the results—positive, negative, and indeterminate—mean.[3] The form should note that the individual has been counseled prior to testing and will be counseled on the results of the test. The form should state that despite efforts to keep the results confidential, test results could become known and reported to state agencies without consent if required by state law.

■ Posttest Counseling

It may be helpful to begin posttest counseling by asking individuals what test result they expect.[3] This gives individuals an opportunity to think about the results and what the impact will have on their life.

Negative Test Result
After informing individuals that the result is negative, assess their feelings. If they are concerned about a false negative, schedule a follow-up test in 3 to 6 months.[2]

Remind all seronegative individuals that if the HIV exposure has occurred recently (eg, the past 6 months) they may not have seroconverted. A follow-up HIV test should be scheduled in 3 to 6 months. Use this time to reiterate the ways that they can protect themselves from HIV infection.

Positive Test Result

The clinician should be prepared for a variety of reactions and emotions after informing individuals that they are seropositive for HIV.[3] Individuals could have feelings of anger, fear, guilt, denial, or combinations of emotions. They could even become suicidal. Therefore, it is important to let individuals have time to discuss their feelings. Some persons, however, will not say anything, and the clinician may have to help elicit their feelings. Some individuals may feel that they are being punished. It is important to let them know that infection with HIV is a consequence of a behavior, not a punishment. Individuals should be asked about support systems[2] and be given information about support groups as well as telephone numbers for the AIDS hot line or a crisis clinic. Some seropositive individuals may worry about social aspects of being HIV positive.[3] It may be helpful for these individuals not to tell anyone except those with whom they have had intimate contact within (at least) the past month. It will also help to reassure them that their HIV test results are confidential.

After individuals have had time to vent their feelings, discuss the meaning of the test results, the virus, and what they can do to take control of what is to follow. Remind individuals that a positive test result means that they are infected and infectious.[2] Measures to prevent them from infecting others must be discussed. Women need to be told of the risk to pregnancy and of delivering an HIV-infected baby. Contraceptives may need to be provided. Discuss with individuals that a positive HIV test does not mean that they have or will develop AIDS.[2,3] It may be between 7 to 11 years before there is any development of disease. Inform infected individuals of the tests used to monitor HIV, such as T4 cell count, and the signs and symptoms of advancing HIV infection.

It may be necessary to arrange more than one posttest counseling visit.[3] Individuals may not be able to absorb all the information at one time. It is helpful to review the information and have them repeat it to ensure that the information they have is correct.

Seropositive individuals must be reminded to tell their partners that they need to be tested.[2,3] This includes those with whom they shared needles and their sexual partners. It may be helpful for individuals to role-play how they will tell their partner(s), or they may want the clinician to help disclose this information. If individuals will not tell their partner(s), try to persuade them to do so. If this does not work, inform seropositive individuals that it may be necessary for the clinician to inform the partner(s). This should be only as a last resort, and in most cases this is not done because of confidentiality issues. However, this could be done with appropriate consent.

Encourage seropositive individuals to begin a healthy life-style by eating properly, exercising, and avoiding substances such as cigarettes and illicit drugs.[3] Alcohol may also affect their judgment on safe sexual practices.

Encourage them to join a support group for long-term support.[2,3]

References

1. Centers for Disease Control. Public health service guidelines for counseling and antibody testing to prevent HIV infection and AIDS. *MMWR.* 1987;36:509–515.
2. Kassler WJ, Wu AW. Addressing HIV infection in office practice. *Primary Care.* 1992;19:19–33.

3. Fang CT, Gostin LO, Sandler SG, Schlotterer WL. HIV testing and patient counseling. *Patient Care.* 1989;23: 19–44.

4. Centers for Disease Control and Prevention. Recommendations for HIV testing services for inpatients and outpatients in acute-care hospital settings; and technical guidance on HIV counseling. *MMWR.* 1993; 42(RR-2):1–17.

5. Janssen RS, St. Louis ME, Satten GA, et al. HIV infection among patients in U.S. acute-care hospitals: strategies for the counseling and testing of hospital patients. *N Engl J Med.* 1992;327:445–452.

TREATMENT OF THE PRIMARY INFECTION AND VACCINES

RICHARD D. MUMA, PA-C
RICHARD B. POLLARD, MD

■ Treatment of the Primary Infection

Since the discovery of HIV as the etiologic agent responsible for AIDS, investigations have turned to the identification and clinical testing of agents that are capable of inactivating this virus. Most of these drugs function as inhibitors of reverse transcriptase (an enzyme unique to retroviruses), although some have other modes of action such as inhibitors of protease.

Nucleoside analogues are the most studied group of drugs active against HIV. In this group, zidovudine (AZT or ZDV) is the only approved drug for initial therapy of primary HIV-1 infection. First approved for individuals with severely suppressed immune systems (CD4 levels < 200/mm³ or a history of *P. carinii* pneumonia),[1] AZT has been expanded for use in persons who are either asymptomatic or symptomatic and have CD4 levels less than

$500/mm^3$.[2,3] In the studies leading to its first approval, AZT was shown to decrease mortality and the frequency of opportunistic diseases in patients with AIDS or AIDS-related complex. In more recent studies, which prompted earlier use of AZT, the data showed that AZT can limit the progression of disease in patients with CD4 levels between $200/mm^3$ and $500/mm^3$.[2,3] These data should be carefully considered when prescribing AZT, since the consequences of early and prolonged use as well as the development of resistance remain unknown. Further, AZT has significant side effects including megaloblastic anemia and granulocytopenia, which should be considered when following patients. The frequency of these side effects has been significantly decreased with the lower dosages now commonly prescribed (500 to 600 mg/day). Most experts agree that AZT should be used earlier in the disease, but there is no evidence to suggest that clinicians should be encouraged to use the drug in all HIV-infected individuals.

Other options for HIV treatment include the nucleoside analogues zalcitabine (ddC) and didanosine (ddI). An initial ddC safety and efficacy study conducted by Merigan et al. determined that ddC was effective in reducing circulating p24 (HIV antigen) levels in patients with AIDS and advanced AIDS-related complex.[4] The major side effect of ddC is a peripheral sensory neuropathy that seems to be dose related.[4] Hematopoietic toxicity has rarely been reported.[4]

ddI also has significant activity against HIV, causing reductions in circulating p24 antigen and increases in CD4 levels. The major toxicities of ddI are peripheral sensory neuropathies and pancreatitis. Both seem to be dose related as with ddC. Other less significant toxicities include diarrhea, anemia, increases in uric acid levels, and perhaps seizures and liver function abnormalities. ddI (300 mg twice a day for patients greater than or equal to 75 kg; 200 mg twice a day for patients between 50 and

74 kg; 125 mg twice a day for patients between 35 and 49 kg) has been approved by the Food and Drug Administration for AZT-intolerant patients as well as for patients who no longer appear to be responding to AZT. In a recently completed AZT and ddI study sponsored by the National Institute of Allergy and Infectious Diseases (NIAID) and Bristol-Myers Squibb[5] (the manufacturer of ddI), AZT appeared to be the more effective drug among HIV-infected patients with advanced disease who had not taken AZT previously, whereas ddI appeared to be the more effective drug among those with previous AZT use of at least 8 to 16 weeks. The exact time to switch stable patients maintained on AZT to ddI remains unclear; however, these recent data suggest that patients may well benefit from this alternate therapy.

The combination of ddC with AZT is indicated for treatment of adult patients with advanced HIV infection (CD4 cell count $\leq$ 300 mm^3) who have demonstrated significant clinical or immunologic deterioration.[6] The recommended combination regimen is one 0.750-mg tablet of ddC orally, administered concomitantly with 200 mg of AZT every 8 hours.[6] Additionally, a recent NIAID study suggests that ddC alone is just as effective and safe as ddI in slowing the progression of disease in HIV-infected individuals who no longer benefit from AZT or who are intolerant of its side effects.[7] However, to date, ddC is being prescribed only in combination with AZT. Although many feel that combination therapy should be increasingly utilized, particularly in advanced cases, the exact pattern of use, dosages, and particular combinations to be recommended await the results of ongoing clinical trials.

Two new classes of drugs (non-nucleoside-analogue reverse transcriptase inhibitors): *Tat* inhibitors, which interrupt the HIV-encoded Tat protein, critical for elongation of transcription, and protease inhibitors, which block protease, a necessary component to form virion core structural proteins of GAG (p17, p24, p15, p9, and p6) and the essential enzymes of POL (reverse transcriptase, ribonuclease H, and integrase), have now entered clinical trials.[8] If effective, both will be attractive alternatives in the treatment of the primary infection. In addition, there continues to be interest in combinations of non-nucleoside-analogue reverse transcriptase inhibitors with nucleoside analogues (ie, AZT, ddC, and a protease inhibitor).

■ Vaccines

Although vaccines are being developed and designed to prevent infection with HIV, their prospect for usage in the very near future seems unlikely. The multiple variations in structure of HIV strains may make vaccines impractical. In addition, the virus may spread from cell to cell, making vaccine-induced humoral or cell-mediated immunity unlikely to be able to prevent infection of a susceptible cell.

Early vaccine trials are under way, and one vaccine has been able to prevent infection in a few nonhuman primates. Development of a vaccine will be slow and, if successful, will require at least an additional 5 to 10 years of further research. Therapeutic vaccines utilized in patients already infected with HIV are being tested in humans. Much more information will be required in controlled trials to determine if this approach will prove to have therapeutic benefit.

References

1. Fischl MA, Richman DD, Grieco MH, et al. The efficacy of azidothymadine (AZT) in the treatment of patients with AIDS and AIDS-related complex. *N Engl J Med.* 1987;317:185–191.
2. Fischl MA, Richman DD, Hansen H, et al. The safety and efficacy of zidovudine (AZT) in the treatment of

subjects with mildly symptomatic human immuno-deficiency virus type 1 (HIV) infection: a double-blind, placebo-controlled trial. *Ann Intern Med.* 1990; 112:727–737.

3. Volberding PA, Lagakos SW, Koch MA, et al. Zidovudine in asymptomatic human immunodeficiency virus infection: a controlled trial in persons with fewer than 500 CD4-positive cells per cubic millimeter. *N Engl J Med.* 1990;322:941–949.

4. Merigan TC, Skowron G, Bozette SA, et al. Circulating p24 antigen levels and responses to dideoxycytidine in human immunodeficiency virus (HIV) infections: a phase I and II study. *Ann Intern Med.* 1989;110:189–194.

5. National Institute of Allergy and Infectious Diseases. Relative benefit of ddI and AZT depends on duration of patients' previous AZT use. *News from NIAID.* December 30, 1992.

6. Meng TC, Fischl MA, Boota AH, et al. Combination therapy with zidovudine and dideoxycytidine in patients with advanced human immunodeficiency virus infection. *Ann Intern Med.* 1992;116:13–20.

7. National Institute of Allergy and Infectious Diseases. ddI and ddC show similar benefits in advanced HIV disease: new options for people who cannot take or who no longer benefit from AZT. *News from NIAID.* January 22, 1993.

8. Johnson VA. New developments in antiretroviral drug therapy for HIV infection. In: Volberding P, Jacobson MA, eds. *AIDS Clinical Review 1992.* New York: Marcel Dekker, 1992:69–104.

Chapter Seven

DIAGNOSIS AND TREATMENT OF COMMON INFECTIONS AND MALIGNANCIES

RICHARD D. MUMA, PA-C
MICHAEL J. BORUCKI, MD

■ Introduction

Some of the common signs and symptoms of HIV-infected individuals are not dissimilar to those of other viral infections. These might include recurrent fever, loss of appetite, chronic weight loss, persistent generalized lymphadenopathy, and fatigue. As the disease progresses and the immune system becomes further compromised (ie, decrease in T4 cells), opportunistic infections may occur. If this happens, other symptoms may present such as headaches, blurred vision, shortness of breath, cough, loss of memory, seizures, focal neurologic findings, night sweats, oral lesions, dysphagia, nausea, vomiting, and diarrhea.

■ HIV and Persistent Generalized Lymphadenopathy

As early as 1979 and 1980, with the discovery of HIV, clinicians began observing persistent generalized lymphadenopathy (PGL) in otherwise healthy homosexual men.[1] Today, PGL is defined as palpable lymphadenopathy of 1 cm or greater size involving two or more extrainguinal sites and persisting for more than 3 months in the absence of a concurrent illness or condition other than HIV infection to explain the findings.[2] Recently, PGL has been placed in group "A" of the CDC classification system for HIV infections.[3]

Clinical Manifestations

Lymphadenopathy may either be discovered by the patient or noted during a routine physical exam in an asymptomatic individual.[1] Symptoms such as fatigue, malaise, low-grade fever, and occasional night sweats may accompany the lymphadenopathy in some patients, as well as a sore throat, fever, and myalgias at the onset of PGL or within few months of onset.[1] Lymph nodes are characteristically firm, nontender, and freely mobile, ranging from 1 to 5 cm in size and involving multiple sites such as the cervical, supraclavicular, posterior auricular, submandibular, axillary, occipital, and epitrochlear.[1]

Diagnosis

Before the diagnosis of PGL can be made, a patient must have palpable lymph nodes of 1 cm or greater involving two or more extrainguinal sites and persisting for more than 3 months in the absence of a concurrent illness or condition other than HIV infection.[1]

Treatment

There is no treatment protocol for patients with PGL. The primary consideration is of alternate causes of adenopathy, such as syphilis, toxoplasmosis, hepatitis B, Epstein-Barr virus, cytomegalovirus, drug reactions, histoplasmosis, tuberculosis, and *Cryptococcus*. Routine follow-up every 3 months, accompanied by an evaluation of the immune system (ie, T4/T8 ratio, absolute T4, white blood cell count, hemoglobin/hematocrit, and platelets), is suggested for asymptomatic patients (see Chapter 14). For patients who are symptomatic and showing signs of progression of their HIV infection (ie, decrease in T4) and PGL, further evaluation, depending on the patient's symptoms, may be necessary.

◼ *Pneumocystis carinii* Pneumonia

Pneumocystis is generally accepted as being a protozoan, although others may classify it as a fungus. The incidence of *Pneumocystis* infection is uncertain. Serologic studies show that up to 75% of children develop detectable antibody by two to four years of age. This suggests that although disease caused by *Pneumocystis* is rare, infection may be common. In humans, the disease occurs worldwide in all age groups, either as epidemics in crowded nurseries or as sporadic cases among older children and adults. Epidemics in nurseries, as well as clustering of cases in cancer wards, suggest the possibility of airborne or respiratory spread. Historically, *Pneumocystis carinii* was a significant pathogen primarily in leukemic children.

    Pneumocystis carinii has traditionally been the most important pulmonary pathogen associated with AIDS.[4] Over 65% of patients with AIDS ultimately develop *Pneumocystis carinii* pneumonia (PCP), and each episode carries about a 10% mortality rate.[5] The prognosis is better with an initial episode than with the second and third episode, but this may relate more to advancing immunosuppression than anything else. Thus, it is appropriate to devote considerable attention to the manifestations, diagnosis, and therapy of this process in an effort to decrease the morbidity and mortality that *Pneumocystis* causes in this population.[4]

Despite intense interest in attempting to unravel the biology and pathophysiology of *Pneumocystis,* the clinician remains confronted with several puzzling features of the illness.[4,6–12]

- The organism cannot be reliably cultured.
- Serologic testing is imprecise and insensitive and for diagnostic purposes is not routinely available.
- In vitro models of infection and sensitivity testing are unavailable.
- In AIDS patients, the signs and symptoms of the illness are frequently subtle and indistinct.
- Standard therapies are frequently associated with significant toxicities limiting their usefulness.
- Recurrent episodes of pneumonia are uniquely common in AIDS patients, and simultaneous occurrence with other pulmonary processes, such as pulmonary Kaposi's sarcoma or cytomegalovirus pneumonitis, complicates management of the illness.

Clinical Manifestations

The classic signs and symptoms of *Pneumocystis* pneumonia are either an abnormal lung exam with fever, shortness of breath, nonproductive cough, and dry rales. Alternatively, there may be a subtle, prolonged preclinical course; mild hypoxia, normal chest x-ray film, and fever and cough may be minimal. Investigation of new minor symptoms often leads to early diagnosis.

Typically, the chest x-ray film shows a diffuse interstitial infiltrate, although discrete areas of pneumonia

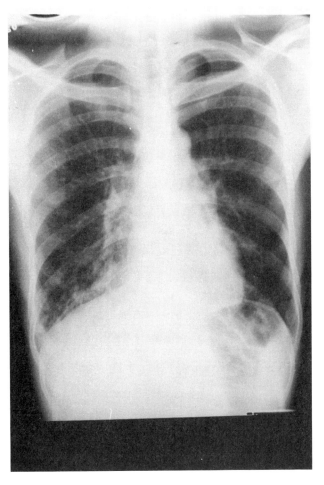

Figure 7–1. Posterior/anterior view of a chest x-ray from a patient with PCP showing diffuse interstitial infiltrates. From *Phys Assist.* 1991;15(2):15,19–22, with permission.

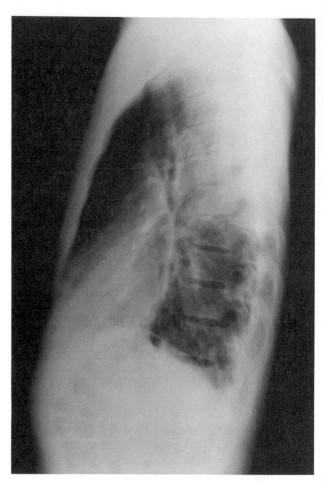

Figure 7–2. Lateral view of a chest x-ray from a patient with PCP showing diffuse interstitial infiltrates. From *Phys Assist.* 1991;15(2):15,19–22, with permission.

may be seen (Fig. 7–1 and Fig. 7–2). The presence of an effusion or of a nodule is sufficiently rare as to suggest an alternate diagnosis. The results of gallium scanning are abnormal in a significant number of cases, even those in which the chest x-ray is normal. However, false positives are common with the gallium scan, occurring in approximately half of the cases.

Diagnosis

The definitive diagnosis of *Pneumocystis* pneumonia is established by demonstrating the presence of organisms. Fiberoptic bronchoscopy is the procedure of choice.[4] Bronchoalveolar lavage via bronchoscopy has nearly 90% sensitivity[4] and significantly less morbidity such that it is the diagnostic of choice. Open-lung biopsy is rarely necessary.

Treatment

Treatment can be initiated with intravenous pentamidine isethionate (4 mg/kg per day) or intravenous trimethoprim and sulfamethoxazole (TMP-SMX; 15 to 20 mg of trimethoprim per kg per day and 75 to 100 mg of sulfamethoxazole per kg per day). The efficacy of these two regimens is similar; there is an 85% or greater rate of response during the first episode and somewhat poorer results for subsequent episodes. The addition of corticosteroid is clearly beneficial in cases where the PO_2 is less than 70 mm Hg or the A-a gradient exceeds 35 mm Hg. Oral atovaquone (750 mg three times a day) is indicated for second-line treatment for mild to moderate cases of PCP in patients who are intolerant to TMP-SMX.[13]

A slow response to therapy is common, and radiographic evidence of improvement may be delayed. The optimal duration of therapy is unclear, but a minimum of 2 weeks for mild disease, and 3 weeks for more severe disease is recommended. Atovaquone is recommended for 21 days. Repeat chest x-ray should be obtained at the beginning of therapy to measure response. Fevers and dyspnea commonly take 5 to 7 days to resolve.

For primary prophylaxis (T4 cells <200/mm^3; presence of constitutional symptoms; without a history of PCP) and secondary prophylaxis (prior history of PCP), it is recommended to use oral TMP-SMX DS, one daily five to seven times a week.[14] For those allergic to TMP-SMX, 300 mg of pentamidine diluted in 6 ml of sterile water administered by a Respigard II nebulizer once a month can be used. Both prevent *Pneumocystis* from recurring, but in a recent study conducted by the AIDS Clinical Trial Group, the investigators found the one-year estimated recurrence rate for the aerosol pentamidine group to be 18.5%, compared with 3.5% for the TMP-SMX group.[14,15] The risk of recurrence in the pentamidine group was 3.25 times that in the TMP-SMX group.[14,15.]

Most drugs have side effects, and pentamidine, TMP-SMX, and atovaquone are no exception. Oral prophylaxis with TMP-SMX tends to be well tolerated, however. Inhaled pentamidine is well tolerated with the exception of bronchospasm in some individuals.

TMP-SMX Toxicities

- Rash
- Fever
- Leukopenia
- Hyponatremia
- Abnormal liver–function tests

Pentamidine Toxicities

- Leukopenia
- Azotemia/kidney failure
- Elevated levels of transaminases
- Dysglycemia
- Hypotension

Atovaquone Toxicities

- Rash
- Nausea
- Diarrhea
- Headache
- Vomiting
- Fever

■ Histoplasmosis

Infection with *Histoplasma capsulatum* has been encountered in many areas of the world but is much more frequent in certain areas such as the United States. Within the United States, infection is more common in the Ohio and Mississippi river valleys and the broad area surrounding them. *Histoplasma* prefers a moist environment to grow, particularly when enriched by droppings from birds and bats. The fungus has been isolated from many sites; one common example is dirt from chicken coops and caves. *Histoplasma* is introduced into the body through inhalation; infection begins in the lungs and can become systemic.

Clinical Manifestations

The vast majority of infections present with a fever of uncertain origin with localizing findings as the infection progresses, or with cough, fever, and malaise. Chest x-ray findings include hilar adenopathy with or without one or more areas of pneumonitis. Acute disseminated histoplasmosis may be mistaken for miliary tuberculosis with severe disease. Common findings include fever, emaciation, hepatosplenomegaly, lymphadenopathy, jaundice, anemia, leukopenia, and thrombocytopenia.

Diagnosis

Serologic tests and clinical manifestations may leave one to suspect histoplasmosis, but definitive diagnosis requires demonstration by culture or histology. In disseminated histoplasmosis, cultures of bone marrow, blood, urine sediment, and biopsy specimens are usually positive.

Treatment

All patients with disseminated or chronic pulmonary histoplasmosis should receive intravenous amphotericin B. The therapy usually takes 10 to 12 weeks and requires doses of 0.4 to 0.6 mg per kg per day. Maintenance therapy is required; however, the optimum doses and duration are unknown for this particular group of patients. Itraconazole (200 mg orally with food daily) for 3 months, or until the infection has resolved, has been approved for *Histoplasma* infections as well. This drug appears to be effective for maintenance, and ongoing studies are investigating the optimal dosing regimen.[16]

Amphotericin B Toxicities

- Decreased renal function
- Hypokalemia
- Thrombocytopenia
- Flushing
- Generalized pain
- Convulsions
- Chills
- Fever
- Phlebitis
- Headache
- Anemia
- Anorexia

Itraconazole Toxicities

- Nausea
- Rash
- Vomiting

■ *Mycobacterium tuberculosis*

Recent reports documented an increased incidence of *Mycobacterium tuberculosis* (TB) among patients with HIV disease, especially those in populations with a high background prevalence of tuberculosis (eg, Haitians, IDUs, inmates of correctional facilities, and economically disadvantaged groups).[17] In the United States there has been an 18% increase in documented cases since 1985.[17] Most people infected with *M. tuberculosis* never develop TB; however, in persons with immunosuppression, like those infected with HIV, TB organisms multiply and cause active disease.[17] Recent reports of multidrug-resistant strains of tuberculosis have complicated this disease, which poses an urgent public health problem.[18]

Clinical Manifestations

Disseminated disease or limited extrapulmonary tuberculosis (especially in the lymph nodes) occurs in 70% to 80% of HIV-infected patients with tuberculosis. Even when the initial presentation involves the lung, an atypical picture is common. Classical upper-lobe apical disease and cavitation are infrequent; the chest x-ray films may reveal only adenopathy or middle-lobe or lower-lobe infiltrates indistinguishable from those produced by other opportunistic infections. Symptoms usually include fever, night sweats, cough, and weight loss, again making the diagnosis of tuberculosis difficult to separate from that of other opportunistic diseases.

Diagnosis

The diagnosis of tuberculosis should be made by bronchoscopy or through biopsy of involved organs. Sputum smear and culture are less helpful because of the often disseminated nature of the disease in HIV-infected individuals but should be obtained. Purified protein derivative (PPD) is also less helpful in the HIV-infected individual because of the decreased ability to react to antigen skin testing in general. However, patients who are HIV-positive and PPD-positive should receive appropriate therapy. Blood cultures are occasionally positive, and new tests (RNA-DNA probes) may allow rapid diagnosis of mycobacterial infection and identification of the species of mycobacteria from a variety of body fluids. Cultures and acid-fast bacillus smears of all suspicious areas should be obtained.

Treatment

The recommended therapy is as follows:

- Isoniazid (INH)—5 to 10 mg/kg per day; usually 300 mg orally daily for 6 months to 12 months and
- Pyridoxine—50 mg orally daily for 6 monthsor as long as INH treatment and
- Rifampin—9 mg/kg per day; usually 600 mg orally daily for 6 months to 12 months and
- Pyrazinamide—25 mg/kg per day orally daily for 2 months.
- For multidrug resistant tuberculosis, five to six drugs are recommended, which include isoniazid, rifampin, pyrazinamide, ethambutol, an aminoglycoside (amikacin, streptomycin, kanamycin, capreomycin), and a quinolone (ciprofloxacin, ofloxacin). The exact drug combination is under investigation and awaits the results of current clinical trials. If a patient presents with resistant strains of TB, an expert in this area should be consulted.

- Isoniazid prophylaxis, 300 mg orally daily for 12 months for all HIV/PPD-positive persons not previously treated.

Isoniazid Toxicity
- Peripheral neuropathy
- Skin rash
- Hepatotoxicity

Rifampin Toxicity
- Hepatotoxicity
- Gastrointestinal
- Fever

Pyrazinamide Toxicity
- Hepatotoxicity
- Fever
- Rash

■ Central Nervous System Toxoplasmosis

The most common cause of focal encephalitis in patients with AIDS is reactivation of a latent infection with *Toxoplasma gondii*. Human infection usually occurs following ingestion of tissue cysts in undercooked or raw meat, organ transplantation, fecally contaminated food, goat's milk, or transmission of trophozoite from mother to fetus in utero.[19,20] The cat is the definitive host for *Toxoplasma*.[21] Infection usually occurs at a young age and lays dormant in individuals with healthy immune systems. However, in patients infected with HIV and a depressed immune system, this protozoan infection becomes reactivated.[21]

Clinical Manifestations

Symptoms range from mild headache and fever to focal neurologic deficits, seizures, and, in some cases, coma.

Extracerebral involvement and coexistent chorioretinitis are occasionally reported.[21]

Diagnosis

The most useful diagnostic test for toxoplasmosis has been the CT scan or MRI. Lesions are usually multiple, ring enhancing with contrast, associated with cerebral edema, and located in cortical or subcortical regions of the brain, such as the basal ganglia.[21,22] Serologic tests are of limited value in the diagnosis of toxoplasmosis in AIDS. Antibody to toxoplasma is prevalent in the general population, and its presence, therefore, has a low predictive value for active infection. Alternatively, very few patients with AIDS and toxoplasmosis are seronegative for toxoplasmosis, so a negative toxo-IgG strongly suggests an alternate etiology. When AIDS patients who are antibody positive are followed prospectively, about 30% of them will develop CNS toxoplasmosis. The clinical and radiologic picture of toxoplasmosis of the central nervous system can be mimicked by several other conditions, including lymphoma, histoplasmosis, nocardiosis, CNS cryptococcus, progressive multifocal leukoencephalopathy, tuberculosis, cytomegalovirus, Kaposi's sarcoma, and hemorrhage.[19,22] Because non-invasive tests lack specificity, definitive diagnosis requires biopsy of the brain, either by open excision or by stereotactically guided needle. However, because of the potential morbidity resulting from brain biopsy and the possibility of false-negative results, some centers favor empirical therapy in patients with positive serologic findings, mass lesions of the CNS, and a clinical picture compatible with toxoplasmosis.[22]

Treatment

Treatment with oral pyrimethamine (200 mg loading dose, then 25 mg per day) and sulfadiazine (100 mg/kg per day up to a maximum of 8 g per day) is usually effective. Folinic acid (5 to 10 mg orally per day) is commonly given in anticipation of megaloblastic anemia[22] caused by pyrimethamine. Clindamycin (450 mg orally every 8 hours) appears to be an effective alternative to sulfadiazine in the sulfa-allergic patient.[22] The optimal duration of therapy is unknown and should be guided by radiographic and clinical evidence of resolution. In most cases, striking clinical and radiographic improvement is apparent within 2 weeks. Pyrimethamine, sulfadiazine, and folinic acid should probably be continued for life. Relapses are frequent, and maintenance therapy, if tolerated, is required. The long half-life of pyrimethamine may make intermittent therapy feasible. One approach is to give 25 mg of pyrimethamine and 2 g of sulfadiazine three to seven times a week.

Pyrimethamine Toxicities

- Skin rash
- Myelosuppression
- Megaloblastic anemia

Sulfadiazine Toxicities

- Renal insufficiency
- Hemolytic anemia
- Agranulocytosis
- Aplastic anemia
- Thrombocytopenia
- Eosinophilia
- Skin rashes
- Liver toxicity

■ Cryptococcal Meningitis

The incidence of cryptococcal infection was rising prior to the beginning of the AIDS epidemic in 1981, presumably because of the increasing use of immunosuppressive therapy in cancer and organ transplantation patients.[23] AIDS, however, has resulted in an alarming acceleration of this trend.[23] *Cryptococcus neoformans* is the causative agent in cryptococcosis, a fungal infection that can become systemic but has a marked predilection for the brain and the meninges.

Clinical Manifestations

The presentation of cryptococcal meningitis in patients with HIV infection ranges from fulminant disease with extensive extraneural involvement to an extremely subtle disease process characterized by mild clinical depression, absence of meningeal signs, and little or no headache and fever.[23] A high index of suspicion and a low threshold for the performance of a lumbar puncture are required for early diagnosis. The less common, fulminant presentation is characterized by multiple sites of involvement (the central nervous system, blood, skin, lung, liver, spleen, and bone) and a rapidly deteriorating clinical course.

Cryptococcal meningitis should be considered in patients who present with any one or more of headache, meningismus, photophobia, mental status changes, seizures, or focal neurological deficits. The diagnosis should also be considered in patients with unexplained fever in the absence of neurological signs and symptoms, and computerized tomographic findings of hydrocephalus or mass lesions should prompt careful evaluation for cryptococcal infection.

Diagnosis

Cerebrospinal fluid (CSF) examination must be performed to exclude the diagnosis.[23] Characteristic findings in patients with cryptococcal meningitis include a mild to moderate lymphocytic pleocytosis, an abnormally elevated protein level, and a depressed glucose level.[24,25] India ink examination of the CSF is positive in a great number of cases and should be performed.[23] Cryptococcal antigen is nearly always detected in the serum and cerebrospinal fluid (of 95% to 100% of cases); therefore, it should always be considered routine. Budding yeast may also be seen on the microscopic exam. Culture of the CSF provides the greatest sensitivity and specificity. However, about 20% of patients will have a normal WBC, glucose, and protein in their CSF, so that diagnosis depends upon cryptococcal antigen and cultures.

Treatment

One treatment regimen for cryptococcal infections is amphotericin B. The optimal dosage and duration of therapy for cryptococcal disease in patients with AIDS are uncertain. Most patients receive a total of 1.5 to 2.0 g of amphotericin B intravenously over at least 6 weeks (0.4 to 0.6 mg/kg per day), but various factors, such as the speed of clinical response and drug toxicity, may influence decisions about therapy.

Therapy with amphotericin B is not curative, and relapse occurs in more than half the patients. Some authorities recommend concomitant therapy with 5-flucytosine. A newer oral antifungal agent, fluconazole[26,27] (400 mg/day orally), has been approved for both the acute and chronic infection. The overall response rate is essentially equal to that with amphotericin B. Fluconazole can be given 400 mg IV once a day for the acute infection as well. The same dose will need to be continued to prevent relapse, and fluconazole is preferred.

Amphotericin B Toxicities

- Decreased renal function
- Hypokalemia
- Thrombocytopenia

- Flushing
- Generalized pain
- Convulsions
- Chills
- Fever
- Phlebitis
- Headache
- Anemia
- Anorexia

Fluconazole Toxicities

- Nausea
- Headache
- Skin rash
- Vomiting
- Abdominal pain
- Diarrhea
- Elevated transaminases

■ Primary Brain Lymphoma

Primary brain lymphoma was one of the first malignancies to be associated with AIDS.[28] It frequently consists of undifferentiated lymphomas of the relatively rare "Burkitt's-like" type (working formulation: small cell, non-cleaved). Primary brain lymphomas have a younger age distribution, there is a very high frequency of extranodal involvement, and the prognosis is extremely poor.

Clinical Manifestations

Like other intracranial mass lesions, primary CNS lymphomas commonly produce focal neurological signs and symptoms (Table 7–1). Hemiparesis, aphasia, and convulsions are usually attributable to supratentorial lesions. Although uncommon initially, seizures occur in patients at some point in illness. Clinical signs of meningeal in-

TABLE 7–1. SYMPTOMS AND SIGNS OF PRIMARY BRAIN LYMPHOMA

Confusion, lethargy, memory loss
Hemiparesis, aphasia
Seizures
Cranial nerve palsy
Headache

volvement are uncommon; their presence should alert the clinician to other causes, such as meningitis from opportunistic pathogens or meningeal metastasis from systemic lymphoma. Confusion, lethargy, and memory loss suggest dysfunction of both cerebral hemispheres and are frequently caused by brain edema, bilateral tumor infiltration, or a coexisting disease.

Primary CNS lymphomas in AIDS patients generally follow a more fulminant course than is seen in immunocompetent patients. In a few reported cases, the clinical progression was extraordinarily rapid, and severe neurological deficits developed over several days. Commonly, neurological symptoms precede the diagnosis of AIDS. One should be highly suspicious of CNS lymphoma when evaluating neurological symptoms in patients with risk factors for AIDS who do not have other manifestations of the syndrome.

Diagnosis

In order to make a definitive diagnosis, tissue must be obtained. Biopsy of a suspected primary brain lymphoma is at times difficult and often leads to inconclusive results. CT scans also can be useful in determining the diagnosis. Although the radiographic findings are variable, intraparenchymal lesions almost always intensify after intravenous administration of contrast material. The enhancement is usually nodular or patchy, although ring and periventricular enhancement patterns have been seen in a number of cases. When lumbar puncture can be safely performed, cytological examination of CSF is a relatively noninvasive method for establishing the diagnosis; however, it lacks sensitivity, as malignant cells are not frequently present in the CSF.

Treatment

Treatment data on primary CNS lymphoma are more extensive for patients without AIDS. Left untreated, the disease is rapidly fatal, and long-term survival is rare. Radiation therapy has been used in a number of patients with some success; however, relapses are very common. The role of adjuvant chemotherapy is unknown. Chemotherapy has not been used to treat AIDS-related malignancies, in a number of cases, because of uncertainty about its effectiveness against primary CNS lymphoma and concern over producing further immunosuppression.

■ AIDS Dementia Complex

As we have seen, AIDS patients are susceptible to a variety of opportunistic infections and neoplasms of the central nervous system. These patients may also develop a subacute or, more commonly, a chronic progressive CNS disorder characterized by cognitive, motor, and behavioral dysfunction.[29,30] Indeed, this disorder, which the medical community has named AIDS dementia complex (ADC), is by far the most common CNS complication in persons with AIDS. ADC is a unique clinical syndrome with a distinct spectrum of underlying neuropathology. Growing evidence suggests that rather than being a sequela of immunosuppression, ADC is probably caused by infection of the brain with HIV.[30,31]

ADC is a clinical term that is largely synonymous with, or incorporates, earlier designations, such as subacute encephalitis or encephalopathy, AIDS dementia, and AIDS encephalopathy. Although ADC may develop before any of the systemic complications initially used by the CDC to define AIDS, it occurs principally in patients already diagnosed with AIDS and is accompanied by morbidity comparable to that of other AIDS-related illnesses. The current CDC definition recognizes ADC as a criterion for AIDS. Dementia is included in the term because cognitive impairment is the most notable and most disabling aspect of the disorder.[31] The word *complex* is included because other neurological manifestations, such as organic psychosis or progressive paraparesis related to myelopathy, are also prominent features that may dominate the clinical presentation and course.[31]

Clinical Manifestations

The clinical features of ADC are sufficiently uniform to allow the definition of a distinct clinical syndrome (Table 7–2).[31–34]

Diagnosis

Neurodiagnostic studies are useful for ruling out neurological complications and for supporting the diagnosis of ADC. They also may provide insight into some aspects of the pathobiology of the disease. The characteristic neuroradiological findings in patients with ADC are listed in Table 7–2.

Treatment

At present, the treatment of ADC is limited to the management of symptoms. Antiretroviral therapy has been introduced for AIDS, and there is some evidence that such treatment helps ameliorate ADC. Zidovudine (200 mg every 4 hours while awake) benefits some patients with ADC. This drug penetrates relatively well into the brain and holds promise of retarding CNS infection.

TABLE 7–2. AIDS DEMENTIA COMPLEX: CLINICAL ASPECTS

Symptoms

Cognitive

Poor concentration, forgetfulness, slowness

Motor

Loss of balance, clumsiness, leg weakness

Behavioral

Apathy, reduced spontaneity, social withdrawal

Signs

Mental status

Inattention, psychomotor slowing, impairment of processing; global dementia, mutism, organic psychosis

Motor findings

Impaired rapid movements, ataxia, tremor, hypertonia, paraparesis, incontinence, myoclonus

Neuropsychological test profile

Impaired sequential, alternation problem solving and complex sequencing

Slow verbal fluency and fine motor control

Overall character

Subcortical dementia with diffuse cognitive deficit, psychomotor slowing, motor impairment, behavioral apathy

Neuroradiological findings

CT and MRI of the head—cerebral atrophy (Fig. 7–3)

EEG—slowing of brain wave activity

■ Cytomegalovirus

Cytomegalovirus (CMV) is infectious for humans of all ages beginning with the gestation period. First called salivary gland virus after it was found to cause subclinical salivary gland infection as well as a fatal, disseminated cytomegalic inclusion disease in newborn infants, it has subsequently been shown to cause a wide spectrum of diseases including congenital malformations, a mono-

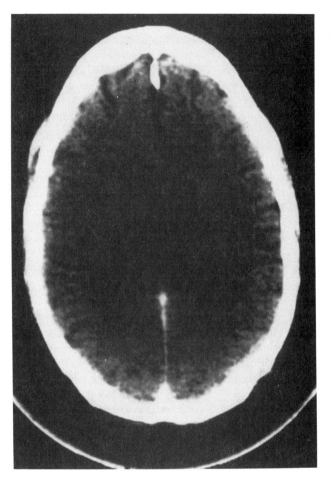

Figure 7–3. Computed tomography of the brain demonstrating cerebral atrophy, a common finding with advanced AIDS dementia complex. From *Phys Assist*. 1991;15(2):15,19–22, with permission.

nucleosis syndrome in adolescents and young adults, and fatal disseminated infection in immunocompromised patients. The name refers to the characteristic enlargement of infected cells. Infection usually occurs after close and prolonged contact, and evidence suggests that cytomegalovirus may be sexually transmitted. The virus has been isolated in saliva, semen, urine, cervical secretions, and feces. Primary infection may also occur after exposure to fresh blood or blood products. Cytomegalovirus infection in AIDS patients can occur as a new infection or more commonly through reactivation of latent virus obtained earlier in life. Approximately 50% to 70% of U.S. adults are CMV seropositive.

Cytomegalovirus belongs to the herpes virus group of double-stranded DNA viruses. It produces large intranuclear and smaller cytoplasmic inclusions in infected cells. The intranuclear inclusions are typically central and surrounded by a clear halo, producing the characteristic "owl's eye" appearance. Cytomegalovirus is a major cause of dysfunction in a wide variety of organs in patients with AIDS. Since cytomegalovirus is so common as a latent virus in the general population, and since cell-mediated immunity is the important element in host defense for controlling its proliferation, it is not surprising that it is a major pathogen. The most common areas affected by cytomegalovirus include the retina, lung, gastrointestinal tract, and, less frequently, the liver. Up to 20% of patients with AIDS may develop CMV disease, and CMV is the most common cause of blindness in AIDS.

Clinical Manifestations

Patients may have fever, weight loss, and severe malaise with primary infection but may complain of shortness of breath (CMV pneumonia), diarrhea (CMV colitis), vision changes (CMV retinitis), or even dysphagia (CMV esophagitis), depending on the location of the infection.

Diagnosis

The definitive diagnosis should be made through histo-pathological evidence (ie, showing the presence of cyto-megalovirus inclusion bodies in tissue) and culture. Infection can also be diagnosed by demonstrating a four-fold rise in antibody titer, but serologic studies may be less reliable in patients with AIDS. In the eyes, the classic "crumbled cheese and ketchup" appearance of exudate with heme is diagnostic to a trained observer.

Treatment

Ganciclovir (DHPG or Cytovene), an acyclovir derivative, has been approved for individuals infected with CMV. The initial dosage is 10 mg/kg per day IV divided into two doses for 14 days. Maintenance therapy is required to prevent relapse, and recommended doses are 5 mg/kg per day. Foscarnet, 60 mg/kg IV every 8 hours for 2 to 3 weeks for induction and 120 mg/kg per day IV for maintenance, has also been approved for CMV infections, usually in those who have failed DHPG.[35] The Studies of Ocular Complications of AIDS (SOCA) trial found im-proved survival in patients treated with foscarnet. Indeed, foscarnet may be the best initial treatment for AIDS patients with CMV retinitis who have normal renal function.[35]

Ganciclovir Toxicities

- Myelosuppression
- Rash
- Nausea/vomiting
- Renal insufficiency
- Suppression of spermatogenesis

Foscarnet Toxicities

- Renal dysfunction
- Renal failure

- Seizures
- Tetany
- Hypocalcemia
- Hyperphosphatemia

■ Oral and Esophageal Candidiasis

Candida albicans is the most common causative agent of oral candidiasis. Oral candidiasis (thrush) is a fungal infection that frequently occurs in patients at risk for development of AIDS (see Chapter 17). The presence of oral candidiasis in patients with pre-AIDS has been reported to be highly predictive for the development of the full-blown syndrome.

Clinical Manifestations

Patients with oral and esophageal lesions usually complain of mucosal tenderness, which is expressed as mucositis or odynophagia. Often, the patients will have white "cheesy" intraoral lesions.

Diagnosis

In oral candidiasis the diagnosis is established by the presence of the characteristic white "cheesy" lesions on the tongue or oropharynx. Examinations of gram-stained or wet-mounted mucosal scrapings reveal budding yeast cells and pseudohyphae. In esophageal candidiasis, mucosal ulcerations may be demonstrated by esophagoscope or barium swallow esophograms. A culture of these areas should be obtained along with potassium hydroxide stains for diagnosis.

Treatment

The recommended therapy is as follows:

- Clotrimazole—30 to 50 mg per day for 14 days for oral candidiasis or

- Ketoconazole—200 to 400 mg per day for 14 days for oral candidiasis or
- Fluconazole—200 to 400 mg per day for 21 days for esophageal candidiasis

Maintenance therapy is required, and the usual dose, if using clotrimazole is 30 mg per day for oral candidiasis; if using ketoconazole, it is 200 mg per day for oral candidiasis; if using fluconazole, it is 50 to 200 mg per day for esophageal or oral candidiasis.

Ketoconazole Toxicities
- Nausea and vomiting
- Anorexia
- Headache
- Epigastric pain
- Photophobia
- Thrombocytopenia
- Elevated transaminases

Clotrimazole Toxicities
- Abnormal liver function (elevated SGOT)
- Nausea
- Vomiting

Fluconazole Toxicities
- Nausea
- Headache
- Skin rash
- Vomiting
- Abdominal pain
- Diarrhea
- Elevated transaminases

■ *Cryptosporidium*

Cryptosporidium is a coccidian protozoan belonging to the class sporozoa.[36] This organism is an intracellular parasite usually infecting cells of the intestine and associated glands. *Cryptosporidium* causes acute, self-limiting diarrhea in nonimmunocompromised individuals. In HIV-infected persons, *Cryptosporidium* can cause severe, protracted, and debilitating diarrhea. Less commonly, a more indolent chronic form of diarrhea can been seen. Although symptomatic disease is largely limited to diarrhea, widespread extraintestinal infection with this organism may occur.

Transmission of *Cryptosporidium* from animals to humans is well documented, and animal handlers are known to be at high risk for acquiring the infection.[37] Although it was initially thought to be the primary mode of transmission, it now appears that many humans do not acquire the pathogen from infected animals.[38] Day-care center outbreaks, nosocomial acquisition, and clustering of cases among close contacts appear to be important modes of transmission.

Clinical Manifestations

Cryptosporidial infection in humans is characterized by watery diarrhea, cramping abdominal pain, weight loss, and flatulence.[39] Most patients report exacerbation of diarrhea and abdominal cramps with food ingestion. Nausea, vomiting, myalgia, and malaise may also be present.[39]

Diagnosis

The diagnosis is made by the examination of the stool with the use of acid-fast staining. Multiple stool examinations are needed, because the organisms may be shed intermittently; even intestinal biopsy may occasionally miss the organisms.

Treatment

Effective therapy for diarrhea induced by *Cryptosporidium* is not available, although more than 20 agents have been used. For now, symptomatic relief such as Lomotil is used.

■ *Mycobacterium avium* Complex

The *Mycobacterium avium* complex (MAC) includes both the organisms *Mycobacterium avium* and *Mycobacterium intracellulare,* and sometimes includes *Mycobacterium scrofulaceum,* which are classified as acid-fast, slowly growing bacilli.[40] Until the onset of the AIDS epidemic, infections with MAC were primarily limited to the lungs in patients with underlying pulmonary disease. Other, less frequent manifestations of infection with MAC in persons without AIDS included lymphadenitis, bone and joint infections, and genitourinary tract disease. Disseminated MAC infections rarely were reported prior to 1981. However, with the increasing incidence of AIDS, disseminated MAC infection has become common.[41,42] It is, therefore, important for clinicians caring for patients with AIDS to be familiar with this important disease process associated with AIDS.

MAC includes the most noted nontuberculosis mycobacteria in the environment and has been isolated from a variety of sources including soil, dust, sediments, water, and aerosols.[43,44] For humans, the most likely source of exposure to MAC appears to be contaminated water.[45] In patients with AIDS, MAC involvement of the bowel is often extensive, suggesting that the gastrointestinal tract may be the site of initial infection, with dissemination to other organs occurring thereafter.[46]

Clinical Manifestations

Since patients with AIDS frequently have multiple simultaneous opportunistic infections, it is difficult to determine precisely which symptoms can be attributed to infection with MAC; persistent fever, weakness, malaise, anorexia, weight loss,[47] and diarrhea[40] appear to be the most common. Fever is almost universally present and may be the only symptom. Often the patient will present with fever of unknown origin. Night sweats are also commonly seen. Diarrhea can vary in volume, consistency, and frequency. Although the most frequent presentation is watery, nonbloody diarrhea, MAC can cause colitis as well as malabsorption syndrome. Weight loss can be dramatic, with loss of more than 15% of body weight over several weeks. Patients presenting with a wasting syndrome should be evaluated for the presence of disseminated mycobacterial infection. Other, less frequent manifestations include lymphadenopathy, hepatomegaly, splenomegaly,[40] and cutaneous and oral lesions. Although found in the lung, *M. avium-intracellulare* rarely causes serious pulmonary disease in HIV-infected patients.[40]

Diagnosis

The identification of clinically significant mycobacteria can be achieved within a few hours, once sufficient growth is available, using nonradioactively labeled DNA probes.[48] A definitive laboratory diagnosis of disseminated MAC should take no longer than 4 weeks.[40] Biopsy of the liver, lymph nodes, or bone marrow and culture of the blood can establish the diagnosis. The presence of large numbers of mycobacteria, often with little or no granuloma formation, is striking in cases of infection with these agents. Large foamy macrophage teeming with acid-fast bacilli are often seen. This is to be contrasted with the paucibacillary histological presentation of *M. tuberculosis*. Large numbers of AFB on stains of the bone marrow suggest MAC rather than *M. tuberculosis*.

Treatment

Approved therapy for MAC infection is currently not available. The organism is resistant to most standard antituberculosis agents but frequently is susceptible in vitro to rifabutin, clarithromycin, clofazimine, ciprofloxacin, cycloserine, and amikacin. In some cases, sensitivity to ethambutol is seen. Treatment rarely results in the clearing of mycobacteria, the amelioration of symptoms, or the healing of lesions. Clarithromycin may be the most promising agent for the treatment of MAC. As is the case with many mycobacterial diseases, multiagent therapy to limit the development of resistance, is probably needed, such as clarithromycin 500 to 1000 mg orally twice a day and ethambutol 25 mg/kg orally every day. Oral rifabutin (300 mg every day) is indicated for the prevention of disseminated MAC disease in patients with absolute T4 cell counts less than 200.[49]

References

1. Mathur-Wagh U, Mildvan D. HIV infection and persistent generalized lympadenopathy. In: Wormser GP, Stahl RE, Bottone EJ, eds. *AIDS and Other Manifestations of HIV Infection*. Park Ridge, N.J.: Noyes Publications; 1987:398–407.

2. Centers for Disease Control. Classification system for human T-lymphotropic virus III/lymphadenopathy-associated virus infections. *MMWR*. 1986;35: 334–339.

3. Centers for Disease Control and Prevention. 1993 revised classification system for HIV infection and expanded surveillance case definition for AIDS among adolescents and adults. *MMWR*. 1992;41 (RR-17):1–19.

4. Suffredini AF, Masur H. *Pneumocystis carinii* infection in AIDS. In: Wormser GP, Stahl RE, Bottone EJ, eds. *AIDS and Other Manifestations of HIV Infection*. Park Ridge, N.J.: Noyes Publications; 1987:445–477.

5. Centers for Disease Control. Update: acquired immunodeficiency syndrome (AIDS)—United States *MMWR*. 1986;35:17–21.

6. Cushion MT, Walzer PD. Cultivation of *Pneumocystis carinii* in lung derived cell lines. *J Infect Dis.* 1984;149: 644.

7. Latorre CR, Sulzer AJ, Norman LG. Serial propagation of *Pneumocystis carinii* in cell line culture. *Appl Environ Microbiol.* 1977;33:1204–1206.

8. Pifer LL, Woods D, Hughes WT. Propagation of *Pneumocystis carinii* in Vero cell culture. *Infect Immun.* 1978; 20:66–68.

9. Hughes WT. Serodiagnosis of *Pneumocystis carinii.* *Chest.* 1985;87:700.

10. Kovacs JA, Hiemenz JW, Machner AM, et al. *Pneumocystis carinii* pneumonia: a comparison between patients with the acquired immunodeficiency syndrome and patients with other immunodeficiencies. *Ann Intern Med.* 1984;100:663–671.

11. Wharton JM, Coleman DI, Wofsey CB, et al. Trimethoprim-sulfamethoxazole or pentamidine for *Pneumocystis carinii* pneumonia in the acquired immunodeficiency syndrome: a prospective randomized trial. *Ann Intern Med.* 1986;105:37–44.

12. Stover DE, White DA, Romano PA, et al. Spectrum of pulmonary diseases associated with the acquired immune deficiency syndrome. *Am J Med.* 1985;78:429–437.

13. New Drugs Drug News. New PCP treatment approved: atovaquone. *Phys Assist.* 1993;17:95.

14. Centers for Disease Control. Recommendations for prophylaxis against *Pneumocystis carinii* pneumonia for adults and adolescents infected with human immunodeficiency virus. *MMWR.* 1992;41(RR-4):1–11.

15. Hardy WD, Feinberg J, Finkelstein DM, et al. A controlled trial of trimethoprim-sulfamethoxazole or aerosolized pentamidine for secondary prophylaxis of *Pneumocystis carinii* pneumonia in patients with the acquired immunodeficiency syndrome. *N Engl J Med.* 1992;327:1842–1848.

16. New Drugs Drug News. Systemic antifungal approved: itraconazole. *Phys Assist*. 1992;16:64.

17. Office of Communications. National Institute of Allergy and Infectious Diseases. National Institutes of Health. NIAID Research Agenda for Tuberculosis. December 1992.

18. Centers for Disease Control. National action plan to combat multidrug-resistant tuberculosis. *MMWR*. 1992;41:(RR-11)1–71.

19. Lenox TH, Haverkos HW. Toxoplasmosis in AIDS. In: Wormser GP, Stahl RE, Bottone EJ, eds. *AIDS and Other Manifestations of HIV Infection*. Park Ridge, N.J.: Noyes Publications; 1987:642–654.

20. Sacks JJ, Roberto RR, Brooks WF. Toxoplasmosis infection associated with goat's milk. *JAMA*. 1982;248:1728.

21. Mariuz PR, Luft BJ. Toxoplasmosis encephalitis. In: Volberding P, Jacobson MA, eds. *AIDS Clinical Review 1992*. New York: Marcel Dekker, Inc.; 1992:105–130.

22. Cohn JA, McMeeking A, Cohen W, Jacobs J, Holzman RS. Evaluation of the policy of emperic treatment of suspected Toxoplasmosis encephalitis in patients with acquired immunodeficiency syndrome. *Am J Med*. 1989; 86:521–527.

23. Masci JR. Clinical aspects of cryptococcosis in AIDS. In: Wormser GP, Stahl RE, Bottone EJ, eds. *AIDS and Other Manifestations of HIV Infection*. Park Ridge, N.J.: Noyes Publications; 1987:680–697.

24. Zuger A, Louie E, Holzman RS, et al. Cryptococcal disease in patients with the acquired immunodeficiency syndrome: diagnostic features and treatment. *Ann Intern Med*. 1986;104:234–240.

25. Kovacs, JA, Kovacs AA, Polis M, et al. Cryptococcosis in the acquired immunodeficiency syndrome. *Ann Intern Med*. 1985;103:533–538.

26. Sugar AM, Saunders C. Oral fluconazole as suppressive therapy of disseminated cryptococcosis in pa-

tients with acquired immunodeficiency syndrome. *Am J Med.* 1988;85:481–489.

27. Stern JJ, Hartman BJ, Sharkey, et al. Oral fluconazole therapy for patients with acquired immunodeficiency syndrome and cryptococcosis: experience with 22 patients. *Am J Med.* 1988;85:477–480.

28. Snider WD, Simpson DM, Aronyk KE, et al. Primary lymphoma of the nervous system associated with the acquired immunodeficiency syndrome (Letter). *N Engl J Med.* 1983;308:45.

29. McAllister RH, Harrison JG, Johnson M. HIV and the nervous system. *Br J Hosp Med.* 1988;40:21–26.

30. Rosenblum BC, Levy RM, Bredesen DE, eds. *AIDS and the Nervous System.* New York: Raven Press; 1988:203–219.

31. Price RW, Sidtis J, Rosenblum M. The AIDS dementia complex: some current questions. *Ann Neurol.* 1988;23:527–533.

32. Berger JR. Neurologic complications of human immunodeficiency virus infection: what diagnostic features to look for. *Postgrad Med.* 1987;81:72–79.

33. McArthur JH, Palenicek JC, Bowersox LL. Human immunodeficiency virus and the nervous system. *Nurs Clin North Am.* 1988;23:823–841.

34. Gabuzda DH, Hirsch MS. Neurologic manifestations of infection with human immunodeficiency virus. *Ann Intern Med.* 1987;107:383–391.

35. Jacobson MA. Foscarnet therapy for AIDS-related opportunistic herpesvirus infections. In: Volberding P, Jacobson MA, eds. *AIDS Clinical Review 1992.* New York: Marcel Dekker, Inc.; 1992:173–189.

36. Leger L. Caryospora simplex, coccidie monosporee et la classification des coccidies. *Arch Protistenkd.* 1911;22:71–78.

37. Current WL, Reese NC, Ernst JV, et al. Human cryptosporidiosis in immunocompetent and immuno-

deficient persons: studies of an outbreak and experimental transmission. *N Engl J Med.* 1983;103:256–259.

38. Hunt DA, Shannon R, Palmer SR, et al. Cryptosporidiosis in an urban community. *Br Med J Clin Res.* 1984;289:814–816.

39. Soave R. Cryptosporidiosis in AIDS. In: Wormser GP, Stahl RE, Bottone EJ eds. *AIDS and Other Manifestations of HIV Infection.* Park Ridge, N.J.: Noyes Publications; 1987:713–735.

40. Inderlied CB, Kemper CA. Disseminated *Mycobacterium avium* complex infection. In: Volberding P, Jacobson MA, eds. *AIDS Clinical Review 1992.* New York: Marcel Dekker, Inc.; 1992:131–172.

41. Blaser MJ, Cohn DL. Opportunistic infections in patients with AIDS: clues to the epidemiology of AIDS and the relative virulence of pathogens. *Rev Infect Dis.* 1986;8:21–30.

42. Wallace JM, Hannah JB. *Mycobacterium avium* complex infection in patients with the acquired immunodeficiency syndrome: a clinicopathologic study. *Chest.* 1988;93:926–932.

43. Fry KL, Meissner PS, Falkinham JO. Epidemiology of infection by non-tuberculous mycobacteria VI. Identification and use of epidemiologic markers for studies of *Mycobacterium avium, M. intracellulare,* and *M. scrofulaceum. Am Rev Respir Dis.* 1986;134:39–43.

44. Ichiyama S, Shimokata K, Tsukamara M. The isolation of *Mycobacterium avium* complex from soil, water, and dusts. *Microbiol Immunol.* 1988;32:733–739.

45. DuMoulin GC, Stottmeier KD. Waterborne mycobacteria: an increasing threat to health. *ASM News.* 1986;52:525–529.

46. Damsker B, Bottone EJ. *Mycobacterium avium-Mycobacterium intracellulare* from the intestinal tracts of patients with acquired immunodeficiency syndrome:

concepts regarding acquisition and pathogenesis. *J Infect Dis.* 1985;151:179–181.

47. Modilevsky T, Sattler FR, Barnes PF. Mycobacterial disease in patients with human immunodeficiency virus infection. *Arch Intern Med.* 1989;149:2201–2205.

48. Gonzales R, Hanna BA. Evaluation of Gen-Probe DNA hybridization systems for the identification of *Mycobacterium tuberculosis* and *Mycobacterium avium-intracellulare. Diagn Microbiol Infect Dis.* 1987; 8:69–77.

49. Department of Health and Human Services. Food and Drug Administration. Rifabutin Approval. December 23, 1992.

Chapter Eight

....
....
....
....

HEPATITIS

DAVID P. PAAR, MD

■ Introduction

Five serologically distinct hepatotrophic viruses cause acute viral hepatitis: hepatitis A virus (HAV), hepatitis B virus (HBV), hepatitis C virus (HCV), hepatitis delta virus (HDV), and hepatitis E virus (HEV). Because the mode of transmission of some of these viruses is similar to that of the human immunodeficiency virus type 1 (HIV), some individuals may be coinfected with HIV and one or more of these hepatitis viruses.

Of the five hepatitis viruses, only three (HBV, HCV, and HDV) have been associated with chronic infection, which, in some instances, leads to hepatic inflammation and necrosis, cirrhosis, and ultimately liver failure. Both the pathology induced by these viruses and the therapeutic response to interferon, the most commonly used agent to treat chronic viral hepatitis, are immunologically mediated events. Thus, coinfection with HIV might reasonably be expected to affect not only the natural history of chronic viral hepatitis but also its response to therapy.

This chapter will provide an overview of the five hepatotrophic viruses and will review what is currently known about the interaction of HIV and chronic viral hepatitis.

■ Epidemiology

Hepatitis A virus is spread predominantly by the fecal–oral route. Contaminated water supplies and foodstuffs and common source epidemics have been described. Specific risk factors that have been associated with HAV include contact with another person with hepatitis, male homosexuality, foreign travel, contact with children attending a day-care center, and illicit drug use.[1]

HBV is spread predominantly by the parenteral route. Risk factors include exposure to blood or blood products (transfusions, hemophiliacs, renal dialysis, and oncology ward patients), exposure to contaminated needles and syringes (injecting drug users, health care workers), and multiple sexual contacts. Thus, hemophiliacs, injecting drug users, and gay men are at risk for both HIV and HBV infection.[2]

The risk factors for acquiring HCV infection are the same as for HBV infection; however, sexual transmission occurs less efficiently and less commonly than HBV.[3] In one retrospective serological survey of injecting drug users and gay men, 73% and 16%, respectively, were positive for HCV antibody.[4]

The acquisition of HDV is closely linked to that of HBV infection. HDV is endemic in certain areas, especially the Mediterranean area, the Middle East, and less so in southern Italy and northern Africa. Delta hepatitis is rare in the United States but does occur in injecting drug users and their sexual partners, hemophiliacs, and multiple transfusion recipients. It is uncommon in gay men.[5]

Hepatitis E virus is an enterically transmitted virus that is spread through fecal contamination of drinking water. It has been responsible for large epidemics of acute viral hepatitis in third world countries.[6]

■ Clinical Manifestations

Acute Hepatitis

The clinical course of acute viral hepatitis caused by any of the above viruses can be divided into four phases: incubation period, the preicteric phase, the icteric phase, and convalescence. After an incubation period that varies depending on the type of hepatitis, symptoms of the preicteric phase include malaise, weakness, anorexia, nausea, vomiting, and pain in the right upper quadrant. The icteric phase begins with jaundice and lasts up to 3 weeks. It seems ironic that symptoms begin to abate soon after jaundice appears. During the convalescent phase, symptoms disappear. Only 20% to 50% of cases of viral hepatitis are icteric. The remaining infections are asymptomatic or are associated with inconsequential symptoms.[2]

The major laboratory abnormalities associated with acute viral hepatitis include elevations in the hepatic transaminases and bilirubin. The hepatic transaminases begin to rise during the late incubation period and peak in the early icteric phase. These may increase to greater than 100 times normal. Alkaline phosphatase may increase, but only one to three times normal. Bilirubin may rise to 20 times normal in the icteric phase.[2]

Chronic Hepatitis

Following exposure to HBV, there is a well-defined immunologic response that results in resolution of illness and protective immunity. The first serologic marker of HBV infection is hepatitis B surface antigen (HBsAg), which is a protein found on the surface of the virus particle. This often persists in serum throughout the period of clinical illness. During convalescence, the disappearance of HBsAg and the appearance of antibody directed against HBsAg, anti-HBsAg antibody, mark resolution of the infection. From 5% to 10% of patients with acute HBV infection do not clear HBsAg and become chronically infected.[2]

Chronic HBV infection leads to either chronic persistent hepatitis (CPH) or chronic active hepatitis (CAH). Both are characterized by asymptomatic periods and periods of disease exacerbation during which fatigue, low-grade fever, right upper quadrant pain, and abnormalities in hepatic transaminases and bilirubin occur.[7]

Chronic persistent and chronic active hepatitis can be distinguished histopathologically. Chronic persistent hepatitis is characterized by mild inflammation in portal triads and hepatic lobules, but there is little or no hepatocyte necrosis. Chronic active hepatitis, on the other hand, is associated with more extensive inflammatory infiltration of portal triads and hepatic lobules. In addition, there is necrosis of hepatocytes at the junction of portal triads and hepatic lobules and extension of necrosis throughout the lobules. The final result of hepatocyte necrosis is cirrhosis, the replacement of necrotic hepatocytes with fibrous material. It is estimated that cirrhosis occurs in 2.5% of patients with chronic HBV infection.[7]

How coinfection with HIV affects the course of acute and chronic HBV infection is currently a matter of active investigation. In one serologic survey of patients with HIV infection, the prevalence of HBsAg was more than twice as great in the group with AIDS as compared to the group with HIV infection but no AIDS. This suggests that advanced immunosuppression may make it less likely for patients to clear HBV infection or more likely to reactivate latent infection.[8]

In another study, the histological and immuno-histochemical characteristics of HBV infection were compared in a group of 20 men with HIV infection and a group of 30 men without HIV infection. Although the liver biopsies of the men with HIV infection had less inflammation and necrosis, there was greater tissue expression of HBeAg and HBV DNA polymerase, indicating that HBV replication was greater in patients coinfected with HIV. It was postulated that the lower level of inflammation and necrosis reflected impaired cytotoxic T-lymphocyte activity, a function that is impaired in those with HIV infection and that appears responsible for hepatocyte destruction in patients with chronic HBV infection.[9] Whether the greater degree of viral replication ultimately leads to accelerated hepatic dysfunction remains to be seen.

HCV has a great propensity to cause chronic infection. Fifty percent or more of those affected will develop chronic infection, and up to 25% of these will develop cirrhosis. Chronic HCV infection is one of the most common causes of cirrhosis in the United States. The histopathologic appearance is similar to that of chronic HBV infection.[3] The effect of coinfection with HIV on the course of chronic HCV infection has not been well described.

Hepatitis delta virus (HDV) can only infect people who are HBsAg positive, because the presence of HBV is required in order for HDV to replicate. Acute delta hepatitis occurs in two forms, coinfection and superinfection. In coinfection, there is simultaneous occurrence of acute HBV and acute HDV infection. Acute coinfection is usually self-limited and rarely leads to chronic hepatitis. Superinfection occurs when acute HDV infection occurs in a chronic HBV carrier. Superinfection results in chronic HDV infection in over 80% of cases. Chronic HDV hepatitis is often severe and leads to cirrhosis and other complications.[5] There is some evidence to suggest that coinfection with HIV adversely affects the outcome of HDV infection.[10]

■ Diagnosis

Acute and chronic viral hepatitis can be diagnosed serologically. The following antigens and antibodies are commonly used for diagnosis: HAV IgM and IgG, HBsAg, anti-HBsAg antibody, antihepatitis B core (HBc) IgM and IgG, anti-HCV, and anti-HDV. Serologic assays for HEV antigens and antibodies have been developed, but they are research tools.

The presence of HAV IgM indicates acute infection with HAV; HAV IgG indicates past infection. HBsAg is present during acute infection with HBV, but the time course may be variable. If HBsAg is absent, the presence of anti-HBc IgM indicates acute infection with HBV. Anti-HBsAg antibody and anti-HBc IgG indicate past infection with HBV. The persistence of HBsAg for greater than 6 months along with failure to develop anti-HBsAg defines chronic HBV infection. The presence of anti-HCV indicates past or ongoing infection with HCV.

The diagnosis of acute delta hepatitis may be difficult because antibody appears late and is sometimes short-lived. Acute delta coinfection can be diagnosed when both anti-HDV and anti-HBc IgM are present. Patients with chronic delta hepatitis will have high titers of anti-HDV and persistent HBsAg.

■ Management

Acute Hepatitis

There is no specific therapy for acute viral hepatitis. Supportive therapy including intravenous fluids, antiemetics, mild analgesia, and antipyretics may be necessary in some cases. It may be prudent to stop potentially hepatotoxic medications until transaminase levels approach normal values.

Chronic Hepatitis

Interferon is approved by the United States Food and Drug Administration for the treatment of chronic HBV and HCV infections; it is used as an investigational agent for chronic delta hepatitis. Interferon can only be administered subcutaneously. Side effects include fever, myalgia, fatigue, hair loss, and bone marrow suppression. Only a fraction of patients treated with interferon have a sustained virologic cure. Clearly, more effective agents with fewer side effects are needed.

For chronic HBV infection, alpha interferon, 3 million units subcutaneously daily for 6 months, is recommended. The response rate varies from 25% to 50%. A predictor of poor response is seropositivity for HIV.[11] However, a preliminary communication indicates that up to 33% of patients with chronic HBV infection and HIV infection with CD4 cells greater than 400 cells/ml respond to therapy.[12]

A nucleoside analogue, fialuridine, which is available as an oral preparation, has been used to treat HIV-infected and uninfected patients with chronic HBV. Although long-term follow-up is not yet available for all patients, the current data indicate that HBV replication can be inhibited in both groups.[13,14]

Chronic HCV infection can be treated with alpha interferon, 3 million units three times weekly for 6 months. Up to 50% of patients respond with a decline in serum hepatic transaminases and improvement of histopathological abnormalities seen on liver biopsy. Unfortunately, many patients relapse following therapy. The focus of current research is to use larger doses and longer duration of therapy with interferon alone or in combination with other agents in order to prevent relapses from occurring.[15]

The results of one small study of 12 patients with chronic HCV and HIV infections (CD4 cells greater than or equal to 162 mm^3) indicate that patients with HIV infection respond similarly to those without HIV infection.[16]

Di Bisceglie et al.[17] reported the results of a pilot study involving 12 patients with chronic delta hepatitis who were treated with alpha interferon, 5 million units daily subcutaneously, for at least 4 months. Two participants were HIV positive but did not have AIDS. Therapy resulted in a decline in hepatic transaminases in 11 patients. This was accompanied by a decline in serum HDV RNA and HDV antigen in most cases. Following cessation of therapy, all patients relapsed. The course of the two HIV-positive patients was not commented upon, but response was reported in 11 of 12 patients, so at least one of the HIV-infected patients responded. Current trials are focusing on long-term and permanent therapy with interferon for patients who have delta hepatitis.

■ Summary

There are five hepatotrophic viruses that cause acute viral hepatitis. Of these, HBV, HCV, and HDV may lead to chronic viral hepatitis. These three viruses occur in patients who are coinfected with HIV. The available evidence suggests that coinfection with HIV may have an adverse effect on the course of chronic viral hepatitis, although more data are clearly needed to substantiate this statement. Presently, interferon is the main therapy for chronic viral hepatitis. Some reports indicate that interferon is equally efficacious in HIV-infected and uninfected patients with chronic HBV and HCV infections, although others suggest that HIV infection is a predictor of poor response in patients with chronic HBV infection. More research is needed to define the effect that HIV infection has on the natural history and therapy of chronic viral hepatitis.

References

1. Lemon SM. Type A viral hepatitis: New developments in an old disease. *N Engl J Med.* 1985;313:1059–1067.

2. Hoofnagle JH. Acute viral hepatitis. In: Mandell GL, Douglas RG, Bennett JE, eds. *Principles and Practice of Infectious Diseases.* New York: Churchill Livingstone, Inc.; 1990:1001–1017.

3. Dienstag JL, Alter HJ. Non-A, non-B hepatitis: Evolving epidemiologic and clinical perspective. *Semin Liver Dis.* 1986;6:67–81.

4. Tor J, Llibre JM, Carbonell M, et al. Sexual transmission of hepatitis C virus and its relation with hepatitis B virus and HIV. *Br Med J.* 1990;301:1130–1133.

5. Hoofnagle JH. Type D (delta) hepatitis. *JAMA.* 1989; 261:1321–1325.

6. Favorov MO, Fields HA, Purdy MA, et al. Serologic identification of hepatitis E virus infections in epidemic and endemic settings. *J Med Virol.* 1992;36:246–250.

7. Hirschman SZ. Chronic hepatitis. In: Mandell GL, Douglas GR, Bennett JE, eds. *Principles and Practice of Infectious Diseases.* New York: Churchill Livingstone, Inc.; 1990:1017–1024.

8. Scharschmidt BF, Held MJ, Hollander HH, et al. Hepatitis B in patients with HIV infection: Relationship to AIDS and patient survival. *Ann Intern Med.* 1992;117: 837–838.

9. Goldin RD, Fish DE, Hay A, et al. Histological and immunohistochemical study of hepatitis B virus in human immunodeficiency virus infection. *J Clin Pathol.* 1990;43:203–205.

10. Novick DM, Farci P, Croxson TS, et al. Hepatitis D virus and human immunodeficiency virus antibodies in parenteral drug abusers who are hepatitis B surface antigen positive. *J Infect Dis.* 1988;158:795–803.

11. Thomas HC, Karayiannis P, Brook G. Treatment of hepatitis B virus infection with interferon: Factors predicting response to interferon. *J Hepatol.* 1991;13: S4–S7.

12. Carreno V, Quiroga JA. Treatment of chronic hepatitis B with alpha-interferon: Present and future. *J Hepatol.* 1991;13:S2.

13. Paar DP, Hooton TM, Smiles KA, et al. The effect of FIAU on chronic hepatitis B virus (HBV) infection in HIV-infected subjects (ACTG 122b). In: *Program and Abstracts of the 32nd Interscience Conference on Antimicrobial Agents and Chemotherapy.* 1992: 264.

14. Fried MW, Di Bisceglie AM, Straus SE, et al. FIAU, a new oral anti-viral agent, profoundly inhibits HBV DNA in patients with chronic hepatitis B. *Hepatology.* 1992;16:127A.

15. Hoofnagle JH, Di Bisceglie AM. Treatment of chronic type C hepatitis with alpha interferon. *Semin Liver Dis.* 1989;9:259–263.

16. Boyer N, Marcellin P, Degott C, et al. Recombinant interferon-alpha for chronic hepatitis C in patients positive for antibody to human immunodeficiency virus. *J Infect Dis.* 1992;165:723–726.

17. Di Bisceglie AM, Martin P, Lisker-Melman M, et al. Therapy of chronic delta hepatitis with interferon alfa-2b. *J Hepatol.* 1990;11:S151–S154.

Chapter Nine

SYPHILIS

STEPHEN G. HAUSRATH, MD

It is no surprise that HIV infection and syphilis are partnered. They are both commonly transmitted in the same way, and actually, syphilis is the easier of the two to transmit or receive. There are epidemiologic data linking them closely, showing that HIV's transmissibility is enhanced when the chancre of syphilis is present. This section is an attempt to describe the diagnosis and treatment of syphilis in a patient with HIV infection.

Syphilis, the many and varied presentations, are caused by the spirochete *Treponema pallidum.* It is restricted to humans and has been described since the days of Columbus. It has long been termed "the great mimicker," meaning that the clinical manifestations are many and, unfortunately, almost never specific. The diagnosis is almost always presumed rather than proved, simply because the organism cannot be cultivated in vitro.

◼ Clinical Manifestations

Primary Syphilis

Usually obtained through sexual contact, the organism invades the bloodstream through mucous membranes or abraded skin. Typically, the site of entry will develop a small raised papule (never a vesicle) that quickly erodes to develop into an ulcer. It usually has thickened borders and appears quite clean. It is described as painless, but this is not universal. Many reports of multiple lesions occurring in patients with HIV infection are available now. This initial infection occurs over a period of days. The actual incubation period is not known in patients infected with HIV but is believed to be as short as 3 days or as long as 90 days. The duration of these lesions is also not really known in HIV-infected patients, but it can be prolonged. These lesions are highly infectious, and a diagnosis can be made directly with a dark-field microscopic evaluation of a scraping. The characteristic, small, helical organisms should be easily seen.

This phase of the disease is called primary syphilis. It is important to understand that although the clinical disease at this point is localized, the organism is by this time widespread, carried through the bloodstream to virtually all parts of the body. Treated or untreated, these lesions of primary syphilis heal. There may be regional lymphadenopathy, but it is not usually tender. It does not suppurate, as the lymphadenopathy associated with the painful ulcer of chancroid will. Clinically, the patient will have no signs or symptoms of any syphilitic disease. The host defenses will develop a humoral antibody response. Although case reports of HIV-infected patients without serologic evidence of syphilis but showing various signs of disease have been published, it appears this is a very rare occurrence. This clinically silent time is referred to as latent syphilis. In the pre-AIDS era, patients who were either inadequately treated or whose immune defenses failed to contain the disease progressed then to secondary syphilis.

Secondary Syphilis

Secondary syphilis is a clinically apparent phase involving the skin. The rash usually develops first on the trunk and then becomes diffuse. An important aspect is that it very often involves the palms and soles. The most characteristic rash is a pigmented macular eruption, although it may be papular or even sometimes pustular. Importantly, it is never vesicular. The organism is present in these lesions, and they are infectious. More often than not, the patient will have additional features of the infection such as fever, weight loss, and malaise. By the time of the development of the rash, the patient will have serologic evidence of infection. Again, rare cases without this are described but are not the rule. The diagnosis then is not usually difficult to make given the characteristic appearance and distribution of the rash and serologic evidence of syphilis. In questioning the patient, however, a history of primary syphilis, or chancre, will not always be obtained. In some patients the initial infection may have been so trivial as to have come and gone unnoticed. It is not clear whether or not HIV-infected patients if untreated will pass through this phase, as every time it is brought to medical attention they are treated. If untreated, it can progress to a fulminant and fatal infection. What does seem clear is that not all patients develop secondary syphilis.

Latent Syphilis

The literature and the textbooks separate two phases of latent syphilis: early latent and late latent. Early latent syphilis describes the silent period during which recurrences of the skin and mucous membrane lesions are likely to recur. In the pre-AIDS era, this was thought of as 1 to 4 years from the time the rash of secondary syphilis developed. Late latent syphilis was then described as the longer period that follows, when recurrences of the dermatologic features were not likely. These terms may not apply to HIV-infected patients. It has been clearly shown now that the progression of the stages of syphilis is altered when HIV is present. The symptomatic periods can be prolonged and the silent periods abbreviated. Put simply, HIV-infected patients can progress rapidly through these stages, and secondary syphilis may never be manifested. There may even be recurrences of what appear to be primary syphilis. It is probably then prudent to describe the clinically silent but serologically evident state as simply latent syphilis.

Tertiary Syphilis

Tertiary syphilis designates clinically apparent disease. Most often this is a neurologic manifestation, but not always. There are case reports of syphilitic arthritis, hepatitis, splenic abscesses, and, in the pre-AIDS era, tertiary syphilis included the cardiovascular manifestations of aortitis and luetic aneurysm. This term, tertiary syphilis, is not specific or very descriptive. It is meant to define a patient with a long exposure to the organism, and the development of advanced disease. It is much more useful now to specifically describe the clinical manifestations in an HIV-infected patient, which more often than not will be neurologic. This simplification must be guarded, however, with the understanding that the less common and sometimes unusual presentations will be found sometimes. It still may be called "the great mimicker."

Neurosyphilis

Neurosyphilis, a specific form of tertiary syphilis, indicates disease of the central nervous system caused by the treponeme. Traditionally there were features of neurosyphilis that were thought of as occurring earlier, and features that occurred later. Again, these temporal descriptions have broken down in the HIV epidemic, and any of the neurologic manifestations are best simply described as neurosyphilis. There may be features of meningitis, encephalitis, or of parenchymal lesions of the spinal cord. The organism produces a vasculitis, and the result may be inflammation, hemorrhage, or infarction. In addition, primary neuronal destruction also occurs. In reviewing a series of surveys, the common symptoms often were mental status changes, seizures, visual disturbances, cranial nerve palsies (including decreased hearing), and motor abnormalities, specifically hemiparesis. In older reports (pre-AIDS), features of ataxias, gait disturbances, and bladder and bowel incontinence are discussed. Tabes dorsalis specifically refers to the loss of neurons in the dorsal columns, and is characterized by "lightning-like" shooting pains and the loss of sensation and proprioception, usually in the lower limbs. Physical findings of neurosyphilis include abnormal fundi, sometimes with papilledema or findings of optic neuritis, abnormal pupillary reflexes, specifically irregular small pupils (the Argyll-Robertson pupils) that react poorly to light but will constrict in accommodation, and the various motor, sensory, or cognitive findings mentioned above.

■ Diagnosis

Above all, a high index of suspicion is needed to bring together the presenting symptoms, physical evidence, and serologic findings necessary to accurately diagnose syphilis.

Primary syphilis is usually evident if complained of and can best be diagnosed with confidence through the use of the dark-field microscopic evaluation of a scraping of the lesion. Generally, most patients will have serologic evidence of disease, but in HIV-infected patients this is not always going to be the case.

Secondary syphilis in its classic form as described earlier should also be easily diagnosed. A full-thickness skin biopsy will show characteristic histological features, and special stains very often can demonstrate the presence of the organisms. Serologic assays are invariably positive in secondary syphilis. Some difficulty in diagnosis may occur when the presentation is less than classic. The lesions may be atypical: raised plaques rather than macules, pustular lesions, involvement of the oropharynx may be the prominent site, and the usual involvement of the palms and soles may be absent. Still, the serology and the use of the biopsy should provide sufficient proof of the diagnosis.

Latent syphilis will only be discovered when screening serologic tests return positive. It is imperative to understand that treatment for this phase is always indicated. Although the patient appears asymptomatic, the organisms are present, and the goal of treatment is eradication of this occult infection and the prevention of progression to the manifestations of tertiary syphilis, which in the HIV-infected patient means neurosyphilis.

Neurosyphilis can be diagnosed when a patient presents with positive serology, any of the neurologic findings mentioned above, and abnormal findings of cerebrospinal fluid examination. The presenting complaint may be sudden or indolent, and fever may or may not be present. Surveys have not yet answered whether or not there is a correlation between neurosyphilis and the T4 cell count. Currently the diagnosis should be considered regardless of the stage of HIV infection. Certainly patients have been described with neurosyphilis and no previous history of opportunistic infections. There will be some difficulty diagnosing neurosyphilis with confidence. It is considered always to be present if the CSF Venereal Disease Research Laboratory (VDRL) is positive, regardless of the dilution present. The difficulty arises when HIV-infected patients present with serologies that are positive for syphilis and neurologic findings but the CSF VDRL is negative.

The central nervous system is believed to be involved in at least half of the HIV-infected population. The various pathologic processes possible are numerous even to list here, but the important point is that abnormalities in the cerebrospinal fluid in an HIV-infected patient may be the rule rather than the exception. Therefore, in entertaining a diagnosis of neurosyphilis in an HIV-infected patient with neurologic findings, it is imperative at least to exclude as many of the more common CSF infections as possible. An MRI of the head will be the most useful imaging study, as it is sensitive to the findings of toxoplasmosis, lymphoma, and, most importantly, progressive multifocal leukoencephalopathy. Assaying the CSF for the presence of cryptococcal antigen will effectively rule out cryptococcosis. Bacterial and especially mycobacterial cultures of the CSF will help at least lower the likelihood of these infections, but a skin test for TB and a careful history of previously treated TB are also important. In the end it may be impossible to rule out mycobacteriosis, and the patient may deserve treatment for this as well as neurosyphilis. Last, a diligent search for evidence of cytomegalovirus (CMV) infection should be made. This would include a dilated retinal exam, and blood buffy coat, and urine cultures for cytomegalovirus. Recent surveys have clearly shown that CMV can and does sometimes cause a parenchymal vasculitis with findings essentially indistinguishable from those of neurosyphilis.

Asymptomatic neurosyphilis deserves some special comment here. Because the progression of syphilis is hastened in the HIV-infected patient, the CDC has recommended that all patients with latent syphilis undergo lumbar puncture. When the CSF VDRL is found to be positive, a diagnosis of asymptomatic neurosyphilis is made. That patient should be treated as having neurosyphilis. It is difficult to decide how to manage an asymp-

TABLE 9–1. SEROLOGIC TESTS FOR SYPHILIS

Assay	Significance
Treponemal Assays[a]	
MHA-Tp	Highly sensitive and specific for syphilis.
FTA-ABS	Indicative of prior infection with syphilis. Not useful in monitoring response of therapy. Once reactive, these tests remain reactive for life. Most useful to confirm reactive or weakly reactive non-treponemal assays.
Non-treponemal Assays	
VDRL and RPR	Both generally signify the presence of infection and are titered out. These titers then change with therapy providing evidence of effectiveness.

[a]The treponemal tests are inherently more sensitive. Following treatment, the nontreponemal assays will often become nonreactive, whereas the treponemal assays may persist for life. It is for this reason that the nontreponemal assays can be used to monitor the effectiveness of therapy.

tomatic patient with latent syphilis given a negative CSF VDRL and CSF pleocytosis and/or an elevated CSF protein. At this time no data can be found that give an adequate solution to this problem. The posture of our experience is this: given an HIV-infected patient with serologic evidence of latent syphilis and a normal neurologic exam, if a lumbar puncture is performed, and the CSF VDRL is negative, but other abnormalities are present, a search for the other above-listed causes of the abnormalities is begun. If no other pathology is found, the patient is treated as described for latent syphilis and followed closely, with a repeat lumbar puncture planned in about 6 months. If the serum titers have responded to therapy, and the CSF VDRL remains negative, the patient is only watched. If there has been no response serologically to the treatment, and CSF abnormalities persist, treatment for neurosyphilis would be recommended.

Serologic tests (Table 9–1) used in the diagnosis of syphilis are available in two kinds: tests that detect antibodies directed against the treponeme itself, and tests that detect antibodies directed against a cardiolipin-lecithin antigen. It is simply a fortune of nature that there is a cross-reactivity between the body's immune response to the treponeme and the cardiolipin-lecithin antigen, which is cheaper and much more available than the assays utilizing the treponemal antigens. Both kinds of assays have their special utilities.

■ Treatment

The principle of therapy (Table 9–2) is to deliver enough of the right drug to the right place for long enough to eradi-

TABLE 9–2. TREATMENT OF SYPHILIS[a]

Primary syphilis Secondary syphilis Latent syphilis	2.4 million units of benzathine penicillin IM once a week for 3 consecutive weeks
Asymptomatic neurosyphilis	Ceftriaxone 1g IM or IV each weekday for a total of 14 doses
Symptomatic neurosyphilis	Aqueous penicillin 4 million units IV every 4 hours for 10 days

[a]There is no alternative to penicillin/ceftriaxone for use in HIV-infected patients at this time that can be recommended on the basis of any published experience. In the case of penicillin-allergic patients, skin testing should be done and consideration be given to desensitization. In desperate cases, chloramphenicol might be considered. Tetracyclines and macrolides are not bactericidal and should not be considered. For treatment of pregnant women and children refer to Chapters 13 and 15 for recommendations.

cate any infection. However, antibiotic therapy is not the only factor in clearing the infection. Host responses clearly are involved, and in the course of HIV infection, are always changing. So at this time, no controlled trials of any regimen for any stage of syphilis are available to guide therapy. Retrospective data, anecdotal reports, and expert consensus is combined to offer some guidance. As new information becomes available, these guidelines may change.

References

1. Burgoyne M, Agudelo C, Pisko E. Chronic syphilitic polyarthritis mimicking systemic lupus erythematosus/rheumatoid arthritis as the initial presentation of human immunodeficiency virus infection. *J Rheumatol.* 1992;19:313–315.

2. Glover RA, Piaquadio DJ, Kern S, Cockerell CJ. An unusual presentation of secondary syphilis in a patient with human immunodeficiency virus infection. *Arch Dermatol.* 1992;128:530–534.

3. Rufli T. Syphilis and HIV infection. *Dermatologica.* 1989;179:117–133.

4. Lukehart SA, Hook III EW, Baker-Zander SA, Collier AC, Critchlow CW, Handsfield HH. Invasion of the central nervous system by treponema pallidum: Implication of diagnosis and treatment. *Ann Intern Med.* 1988;109:855–862.

5. Kanda T, Shinohara H, Suzuki T, Murata K. Depressed CD4/CD8 ratio in TPHA-negative patients with syphilis. *Microbiol Immunol.* 1992;36(3):317–320.

6. Imperator PJ. Syphilis, AIDS and crack cocaine. *J Commun Health.* 1992;17(2):69–71.

7. Fabian RH. Neurologic diseases associated with trophic skin lesions. In: Demis DJ, ed. *Clinical Dermatology.* Vol. 4, Unit 29-5, Nineteenth revision. Philadelphia: JB Lippincott; 1992:1–6.

8. Rompalo AM, Cannon RO, Quinn TC, Hook EW III. Association of biologic false-positive reactions for syphilis with human immunodeficiency virus infection. *J Infect Dis.* 1992;165:1124–1126.

9. Marra CM, Handsfield HH, Kuller L, Morton WR, Lukehart SA. Alterations in the course of experimental syphilis associated with concurrent simian immunodeficiency virus infection. *J Infect Dis.* 1992;165: 1020–1025.

10. Hook EW III. Management of syphilis in human immunodeficiency virus-infected patients. *Am J Med.* 1992;93:477–479.

11. Pereira LH, Embil JA, Haase DA, Manley KM. Prevalence of human immunodeficiency virus in the patient population of a sexually transmitted disease clinic. *Sex Transm Dis.* 1992;19:115–120.

12. DiNubile MJ, Baxter JD, Mirsen TR. Acute syphilitic meningitis in a man with seropositivity for human immunodeficiency virus infection and normal numbers of CD4 T lymphocytes. *Arch Intern Med.* 1992; 152:1324–1326.

13. Holtom PA, Larsen RA, Leal ME, Leedom JM. Prevalence of neurosyphilis in human immunodeficiency virus-infected patients with latent syphilis. *Am J Med.* 1992;93:9–12.

14. Dowell ME, Ross PG, Musher DM, Cate TR, Baughn RE. Response of latent syphilis or neurosyphilis to ceftriaxone therapy in persons infected with human immunodeficiency virus. *Am J Med.* 1992;93:481–488.

15. Johns DR, Tierney M, Felsenstein D. Alteration in the natural history of neurosyphilis by concurrent infection with the human immunodeficiency virus. *N Engl J Med.* 1987;316:1569–1572.

16. Katz DA, Berger JR. Neurosyphilis in acquired immunodeficiency syndrome. *Arch Neurol.* 1989;46:895–898.

17. Musher DM, Hamill RJ, Baughn RE. Effect of human immunodeficiency virus (HIV) infection on the course of syphilis and on the response to treatment. *Ann Intern Med.* 1990;113:872–881.

18. Manganoni AM, Graifemberghi S, Facchetti F, Gavazzoni R, DePanfilis G. Effectiveness of penicillin G benzathine therapy for primary and secondary syphilis in HIV infection. *J Am Acad Dermatol.* 1990; 23(1):1185.

19. Mandell GL, Douglas RG, Bennett JE, eds. *Principles and Practice of Infectious Diseases.* 3rd ed. New York: Churchill Livingstone Inc.; 1990.

20. Braude AI, Davis CE, Fierer J, eds. *Infectious Diseases and Medical Microbiology.* 2nd ed. Philadelphia: WB Saunders; 1986.

Chapter Ten

RECOGNITION AND MANAGEMENT OF ADVERSE DRUG REACTIONS

JOHN E. FUCHS, JR., PharmD

■ Introduction

The goal of recommending a drug to a person is to treat a condition without creating a problem. Unfortunately, problems are inevitable occurrences in all populations that receive medications. With certain drugs, however, patients with HIV infection have a greater tendency to develop adverse reactions compared to the non-HIV patient.[1] Additionally, HIV patients may receive numerous medications to treat multiple medical problems. It is known that the greater the number of medications a patient takes, the more likely is the risk of adverse drug reactions. Since it is sometimes difficult to differentiate disease from drug-induced abnormalities, recognizing and managing an adverse reaction in a patient with multiple diseases and medications is a challenge. It is important not to forget that medications can be a problem instead of a solution.

■ Definition

An adverse drug reaction (ADR) is an unintended nuisance or a potentially life-threatening effect of a drug. Adverse drug reactions can be classified as either related or not related to the dose (or serum level) of a drug. Some characteristics of serum-level-related ADRs include improvement upon drug dosage reduction, and they may be predictable. Non-serum-level-related ADRs, such as allergic or hypersensitivity reactions, respond only to drug discontinuation and are considered unpredictable. Sometimes, risk factors can be identified that increase the likelihood of an ADR.

■ Getting Started—Reviewing the Medication Regimen

Many ADRs are predictable from the dose, the serum level, or the number of medications a patient receives. In some cases, ADRs must be accepted, and one hopes they will be mild. However, minimizing the risk or the severity of predictable adverse reactions at each patient visit can be accomplished by reviewing the medication regimen and preventing overmedication. This involves four steps:

1. Discontinuing unnecessary medications (every drug must have an active diagnosis).
2. Determining that each dose is correct for body weight, hepatic, and renal function.
3. Recognizing a sign or symptom as a potential adverse drug reaction.
4. Recognizing potentially significant drug interactions.

■ Recognition

Recognition of an ADR begins with an index of suspicion that a particular sign or symptom is causally related to the use of a drug. Literature-documented ADRs can be helpful in diagnosing the ADR, but not necessarily a requirement. Identifying risk factors is helpful, but is not absolute. Differentiation between ADRs and disease symptomatology is sometimes difficult but can be accomplished by:

1. Determining the onset of the complaint relative to drug use.
2. Identification of risk factors that increase the likelihood of ADR (which can be a concurrent illness).
3. Response to subsequent dose reductions and/or drug discontinuation (and perhaps reintroduction of suspected drug).
4. Ruling out concurrent disease entities with appropriate diagnostic evaluation.

It is not always possible to determine the causal relationship with a drug and the ADR.

A list of previously reported and common adverse drug reactions is found in Table 10–1.

Management

Once the ADR is recognized and is determined to be a nuisance or potentially life threatening, management usually consists of dosage reduction or drug discontinuation. Depending on available alternatives and the severity of the ADR, reintroduction of the drug at a later time could be an option especially if the ADR is dose related. Reintroduction of a drug following a hypersensitive reaction may require a desensitization plan. Management of ADRs depends on:

1. Recognition and differentiation from disease.
2. Assessing severity.
3. Dosage reduction and/or drug discontinuation.
4. Available alternative therapy.
5. Reintroduction of drug after resolution of ADR: lower dose or desensitization.

TABLE 10–1. PREVIOUSLY REPORTED AND COMMON ADVERSE DRUG REACTIONS

Drug	Adverse Effects
Acyclovir	*Intravenous:* thrombophlebitis, confusion, hallucinations, renal impairment, (must be diluted in 100 ml of normal saline and infused over 1 hour)
	Oral: long term (1 to 2 years) rarely causes headache, dizziness, arthralgia
Amphotericin B	Normochromic normocytic anemia, hypokalemia, hypomagnesemia, renal impairment, infusion-related fever and chills
Azithromycin	Abdominal pain
Ciprofloxacin	Rare CNS reactions; rare increased liver function tests; arthropathy (avoid in patients < 18 years old)
Clarithromycin	Nausea, abdominal pain (increase with doses > 1 g/day)
Clofazimine	Nausea, abdominal pain, skin discoloration (pink-brown)
Co-trimoxazole	*Intravenous:* bone marrow suppression, tremor, rash
	Oral: rash, fever, nausea
Dapsone	Peripheral neuropathy, hemolytic anemia
Didanosine	Pancreatitis, peripheral neuropathy
Ethambutol	Peripheral neuropathy, optic neuritis, hyperuricemia, metallic taste
Filgrastim	Bone pain, hyperuricemia, abnormal taste
Fluconazole	Abdominal pain
Flucytosine	Neutropenia, thrombocytopenia, nausea
Foscarnet	Anemia, renal dysfunction, hyperphosphatemia, hypocalcemia (ionized calcium should be monitored)
Ganciclovir	Neutropenia, thrombocytopenia, disorientation with high dose for prolonged periods
Isoniazid	Hepatitis, peripheral neuropathy, drug-induced SLE

TABLE 10–1. (continued)

Adverse Drug Reactions

Drug	Adverse Effects
Itraconazole	Hypertriglyceridemia, hypokalemia (doses > 400 mg/day), adrenal insufficiency (doses > 600 mg/day)
Ketoconazole	Nausea, abdominal pain, hepatitis, hypertriglyceridemia, adrenal suppression (doses > 600 mg/day)
Metronidazole	Peripheral neuropathy (doses > 1500 mg/day)
Pentamidine	*Intravenous:* pancreatitis, neutropenia, hypoglycemia, hypotension, renal insufficiency *Inhalation:* metallic taste, anorexia, bronchospasm, pancreatitis
Pyrazinamide	Hyperuricemia, hepatitis (doses > 30 mg/kg per day), arthralgia
Pyrimethamine	Megaloblastic anemia, neutropenia
Rifampin	Hypersensitive thrombocytopenia and interstitial nephritis, reddish-orange discoloration of urine, stool, saliva, and sweat
Sulfadiazine	Crystalluria and renal failure, rash, neutropenia
Zalcitabine	Peripheral neuropathy, pancreatitis, arthralgia, esophageal and mouth ulcers
Zidovudine	Neutropenia, megaloblastic anemia (bone marrow recovery 14 days), headache, blue nail pigmentation, proximal myopathy of legs associated with increased CPK

Peripheral neuropathy, pancreatitis, renal dysfunction, and neutropenia deserve further attention, as they are more likely to be encountered in clinical practice.

■ Peripheral Neuropathy[3,4]

Comment

HIV, CMV, and vitamin B_{12} deficiencies have been associated with peripheral neuropathies in AIDS patients. Although the etiology of peripheral neuropathy of some drugs is known, such as isoniazid, it is unclear whether other drugs associated with peripheral neuropathy induce or exacerbate existing disease. When a patient develops activity-limiting peripheral neuropathy, it is appropriate to lower dosages or withdraw the suspected neurotoxins to establish a causal relationship.

Drugs

1. Zalcitabine
2. Isoniazid[5]
3. Dapsone
4. Metronidazole
5. Didanosine[6]
6. Ethionamide

Risk Factors for Drug-Induced Peripheral Neuropathy

1. Advancing HIV disease (absolute T4 < 50)
2. Vitamin B_{12} deficiency
3. Previous peripheral neuropathy or concurrent neurotoxin

Recognition

1. Sensory neuropathy is the rule (eg, tingling, numbness, burning, or pain in the feet or hands); motor involvement is rare
2. Reduced or absent achilles reflex

Management
Non-Activity-Limiting

1. Discontinue unnecessary neurotoxin
2. Use lowest effective dose for suspected neurotoxins (both ddI and ddC require dosage reduction in renal insufficiency)
3. Therapeutic trial:
   a. Ibuprofen 400 to 600 mg, 3 doses/day
   b. Amitriptyline/nortriptyline 25 to 50 mg once daily

Activity-Limiting Neuropathy (persistence > 3 days)

1. Reduce dosage or discontinue suspected drug
2. Recovery may take over 2 weeks to several months
3. When symptoms decrease or resolve, reintroduce drug at lower dosage

■ Pancreatitis[7]

Comment

Advancing HIV disease and CMV have been associated with pancreatitis in the absence of drug therapy. When a patient develops clinical pancreatitis, it is appropriate to provide a drug-free period of suspected pancreatoxins to establish the causal relationship.

Drugs

1. Didanosine[8,9]
2. Zalcitabine
3. Ganciclovir
4. Pentamidine (intravenous)[10]
5. Pentamidine (inhalation)[11]

Risk Factors for Drug-Induced Pancreatitis

1. Concurrent alcohol consumption
2. Hypertriglyceridemia
3. Previous pancreatitis
4. Absolute CD4 lymphocyte less than 50

Recognition

1. Abdominal pain, nausea, and vomiting; associated with elevations in amylase, lipase enzymes, or both
2. Hypocalcemia
3. Hypertriglyceridemia

Management

1. Correct dosages for renal insufficiency.
2. Encourage patient to discontinue alcohol ingestion.
3. Asymptomatic elevations in pancreatic enzymes are more common than symptomatic pancreatitis. However, if salivary fraction of amylase has been ruled out, suspected pancreatoxins should be discontinued if enzyme(s) exceed four times the upper limit of normal to determine causal relationship.
4. Discontinue suspected pancreatoxin if patient is symptomatic and pancreatic enzymes are two times upper limit of normal to determine causal relationship.
5. When pancreatic enzymes have normalized, rechallenge with reduced dosage and repeat enzymes in 5 to 7 days if alternative therapy is unavailable.

■ Renal Dysfunction

Comment

An HIV nephropathy that usually leads to renal failure has been described, but drugs are the most common cause of renal dysfunction. Recovery from drug-induced lost renal function is the rule when the nephrotoxin is discontinued.

Drugs

1. Amphotericin B*[12]
2. Foscarnet
3. Pentamidine (intravenous)
4. Acyclovir (intravenous)
5. Sulfadiazine[13]

Risk Factors for Drug-Induced Renal Dysfunction

1. Dehydration†
2. Hyponatremia
3. Concurrent nephrotoxins‡

Recognition

1. Recent elevation of serum creatinine above upper limits of normal
2. Impaired urinary concentrating ability
3. Proteinuria
4. Urinary casts

Management

1. Correct dosage for renal dysfunction.
2. Correct dehydration/hyponatremia; infuse 500 to 1000 ml normal saline, then 2 to 3 liters per day.

---

*Renal tubular acidosis produces reduced GFR, hypokalemia, hypomagnesemia, and hyponatremia; may take several months after amphotericin is discontinued to normalize.

†Increase dietary sodium intake and/or infuse 500 to 2000 ml normal saline.

‡Aminoglycosides, vancomycin.

---

3. If rehydration is insufficient, reduce dosage appropriately or discontinue until serum creatinine has normalized.

■ Neutropenia[14,15]

Comment

Neutropenia predisposes a patient to infection. It is estimated that 20% to 25% of patients with HIV infections have low circulating neutrophils, but neutrophil function may also be impaired (eg, chemotaxis, phagocytosis, and killing power). When a patient develops neutropenia, it is appropriate to lower the dosage, or withdraw the suspected bone marrow suppressant, or administer a neutrophilic hematopoietic factor to prevent a life-threatening infection. Hematopoietic factors may allow continuation of bone marrow suppressant.

Drugs

1. Zidovudine
2. Ganciclovir
3. Flucytosine
4. Pyrimethamine
5. Pentamidine
6. Sulfonamides

Risk Factors

Concurrent bone marrow-suppressing agents

Recognition

Absolute granulocyte count (ANC) less than 750 cells/ mm^3 (total WBC × [% segs + % bands]).

Management

1. Correct dosage for body weight and renal function.
2. Withdraw suspected agent, if considered unnecessary.
3. If bone marrow suppressant cannot be discontinued, administer filgrastim (gCSF), 5 μg/kg* subcutaneously or intravenously once daily for three to four consecutive days. Maintenance dose will likely be 5 μg/kg, one to three times weekly†

NOTE: Target ANC is 1500 cells/mm^3. Discontinue filgrastim if ANC is above 15,000 cells/mm^3‡

References

1. Kovacs JA, Hiemenz JW, Macher AM, et al. *Pneumocystis carinii* pneumonia: a comparison between patients with the acquired immunodeficiency syndrome and patients with other immunodeficiencies. *Ann Intern Med.* 1984;100:663–671.
2. McQueen EF. Pharmacological basis of adverse drug reactions. In: Speight TM, ed. *Avery's Drug Treatment: Principles and Practice of Clinical Pharmacology and Therapeutics.* 3rd ed. Baltimore, MD: Williams & Wilkins; 1987:229.
3. Cornblath DR, McArthur JC. Predominant sensory neuropathy in patients with acquired immunodeficiency syndrome and AIDS related complex. *Neurology.* 1988;38:794–796.
4. Simpson DM, Olney RK. Peripheral neuropathy with human immunodeficiency virus infection. *Neurology Clinics.* 1992;10:685–711.

---

*Round off to nearest 50 μg; vial contains 300 μg/ml.
†Monitor CBC weekly.
‡Sargramostim (gmCSF) is an alternative.

---

5. Gibson FD, Phillips S. Peripheral neuritis after long term isoniazid. *Geriatrics.* 1966;21:178–181.

6. Kiebartz KD, Siedlin M, Lambert JS, et al. Extended follow up of peripheral neuropathy in patients with AIDS and ARC treated with didanosine. *J AIDS.* 1992;5:60–64.

7. Schwartz MS, Brandt LJ. The spectrum of pancreatitis disorder in patients with AIDS. *Am J Gastroenterol.* 1989;84:459–462.

8. Rathburn CR, Martin ES. Didanosine therapy in patients intolerant of or failing zidovudine therapy. *Drug Intell Clin Pharm.* 1992; 62:1347–1351.

9. Maxson CJ, Greenfield SM, Turner JL. Acute pancreatitis as a common complication of didanosine in AIDS. *Am J Gastroenterol.* 1992;87:708–713.

10. O'Neil M, Selub SE, Hak LF. Pancreatitis during pentamidine therapy in patients with AIDS. *Clin Pharmacol.* 1991;10:56–59.

11. Murphy RL, Noskin GA, Ehrenpreis ED. Acute pancreatitis associated with inhaled pentamidine. *Am J Med.* 1990;5N:553–556.

12. Heidemann HT, Gerkens JF, Spickard WA, et al. Amphotericin B nephrotoxicity in humans decreased by salt repletion. *Am J Med.* 1983;75:476–481.

13. Simon DI, Brosios FC, Rothstein DM. Sulfadiazine crystalluria revisited. *Arch Intern Med.* 1990;150:2379–2384.

14. Murphy MF, Metcalfe P, Waters AH, et al. Incidence and mechanism of neutropenia and thrombocytopenia in patient with human immunodeficiency virus infection. *Br J Haematol.* 1987;66:337–340.

15. Israel DS, Plaisance KI. Neutropenia in patients infected with human immunodeficiency virus. *Clin Pharmacol.* 1991;10:268–279.

Chapter Eleven

INTERPRETING LABORATORY DATA

JANICE G. CURRY, PA-C

Interpreting lab data of HIV-infected patients is often a challenging, and sometimes frustrating, endeavor. The normal value ranges are generally more variable and may need to be based on the patient's overall disease progression. What may appear to be a panic lab value may be well within a patient's norm, conversely, a "normal" value may represent a significant change from the patient's norm. Two examples are:

1. A white blood cell count of 7.8 in a patient with advanced AIDS who normally has a total white blood cell count of 1.2.
2. Hypocalcemia in a profoundly nutritionally depleted patient with a decreased albumin level.

Questions that should always be foremost in the clinician's mind when interpreting lab data are:

1. Is this a change for this patient or an unexpected abnormality?

2. Is the patient symptomatic? (ie, is the patient with a low hemoglobin/hematocrit having any clinical signs and/or symptoms of anemia?)
3. Could this be a drug-induced abnormality?
4. Does this lab abnormality actually represent an improvement for this patient?
5. How competent is the patient's immune system?
6. Are the lab abnormalities heralding a new opportunistic infection, or are they a manifestation of HIV itself?

If all these factors are evaluated when interpreting data, then therapeutic treatments or additional diagnostic studies will be more appropriately instituted and occasionally avoided. HIV-related processes affect every organ system in the human body; however, it does not follow that every disease or health problem is an HIV-related event. The following is a brief look at some laboratory and diagnostic abnormalities and their possible causes.

■ Establishing the Diagnosis of HIV

A variety of tests are used to establish the diagnosis of HIV. Human immunodeficiency virus can be isolated (or cultured) from concentrated peripheral blood lymphocytes and less frequently from body fluids.[1] However, culture is difficult, expensive, takes several days, is not frequently available in most laboratories, and is positive more often in the early stages of infection than in later stages.[1]

HIV viral antigen may become detectable as soon as 2 weeks after infection and usually lasts roughly 3 to 5 months. New DNA probe kits are commercially available but are not used as a standard test. Eventually antigen detection should most likely be the method of choice to detect infection in the first few weeks after exposure.[1]

The ELISA (enzyme-linked immunosorbent assay) is used most commonly to detect the presence of antibody to HIV. A reactive ELISA is used to diagnose HIV infection indirectly. A positive or reactive ELISA is repeated using the same blood sample. If repeatedly reactive, the Western blot is performed. A positive Western blot is considered a confirmatory test for the presence of antibody to HIV.[2]

Nonreactive HIV test results can occur during the acute stage of infection when the virus is present but an antibody response has not yet developed. This period of time before antibody is detected may be as long as 6 months. During this period, a test for HIV antigen (P24) may suggest HIV infection.[2,3]

There is also controversy whether reactivity against only a single antibody of a certain type (eg, the core proteins GAG p15/p17 or the envelope glycoproteins gp 120/160) is sufficient to consider the test truly reactive and thus indicative of HIV infection in the absence of reactivity against antibodies to more than the single protein. When this happens, it is often considered a false positive or an "indeterminant" reaction, although its significance has not yet been definitely established.[1]

When interpreting tests for HIV, one must remember that a positive test indicating HIV infection does not mean AIDS. AIDS is a clinical diagnosis. HIV infection is the continuum of clinical conditions ranging from the mononucleosis-like syndrome associated with seroconversion through asymptomatic HIV infection to symptomatic HIV infection, and finally to AIDS.[4]

■ Absolute T4 (CD4) Count

A method for following the progression of HIV infection is measurement of the T lymphocytes. Specific laboratory tests include the absolute T4 counts (Table 11–1) and the

TABLE 11–1. THERAPY DECISIONS BASED UPON T4 COUNT AND CLINICAL FEATURES

T4 Values (Normal range 500–1000)	Stage and Clinical Features	Therapy Decisions
1000–500	Acute retroviral syndrome/asymptomatic. Intermittent symptoms, oral candidiasis, oral ulcers, lymphadenopathy, xerosis, rashes (seborrheic dermatitis, folliculitis).	Treat symptomatically
Below 500	Asymptomatic/symptomatic. Chronic or intermittent symptoms. Lymphadenopathy, oral candidiasis, oral lesions, nausea, vomiting, diarrhea, fevers, night sweats, tuberculosis, zoster, *Nocardia*, Kaposi's sarcoma may be seen.	Begin antiretroviral therapy
Below 200	Increasingly severe and persistent symptoms. Memory or cognitive deficits. Life-threatening infections. Increased incidence of cancers and pulmonary and CNS pathology. Increased risk of disseminated disease processes. AIDS defining infections such as PCP, Toxo, Histo, Crypto.	Antiretroviral therapy and prophylaxis (as available) is crucial. Consider change in antiretroviral if immunoclinically failing.
Below 50	Increased/high probabilities of opportunistic infections and mortality, PML, AIDS dementia, CMV, MAI, and other late-stage processes.	According to patient and disease process. Patient should maintain antiretroviral therapy and prophylactic treatments. Consider change in antiretroviral therapy or combination therapy. Potential benefit of MAI prophylaxis.

T4/T8 ratio.[2,5] Although these values do not indicate the patient's current health, they do provide a guide to whether the patient is at a negligible, modest, or marked risk for AIDS-related opportunistic infections. Monitoring T4 counts allows the clinician to predict with increasing accuracy an individual's risk for the development of opportunistic infections, which is directly related to immunodeficiency.[6] The results are also a guide by which antiretroviral therapy and prophylactic treatment decisions can be made.

The T4 count should be drawn at the time of initial evaluation and at a second visit 2 to 6 weeks later to establish a baseline (Table 11–2). Depending on clinical symptoms, T4 counts should be drawn every 2 to 4 months after the base-

TABLE 11–2. T4 VALUES VERSUS INTERVAL FOR FOLLOW-UP

T4 Value	Interval	Reason for Monitoring
> 500 Repeatedly	Every 4 months	Deciding when to institute anti-retroviral therapy
500–200	Every 2 to 3 months	Monitoring response to anti-retroviral therapy and to decide when to initiate prophylaxis for *Pneumocystis* pneumonia
200–50	Every 2 months	Evaluating the need to change antiretroviral therapy, considering other prophylaxis (as available), and assessing the risk for opportunistic infections
<50 Repeatedly	?	Monitoring may only increase patient anxiety

line value has been established.[3,5] Once T4 counts fall below 50, their value in relation to disease progression is somewhat reduced, and procuring additional levels rarely varies treatment. It should also be noted that variations of up to 15% for an individual may be normal.

Other laboratory tests that help in determining how active the virus may be in an individual are the beta-2 microglobulin (B2M) and the p24 antigen.[2,6] These values may be abnormal during active progression of the patient's HIV disease. Serum concentrations of B2M greater than 3 mg/L have been shown to be a predictor of the development of AIDS.[7] Detection of p24 antigen, one of the core proteins, in the serum of an HIV-positive person appears to reflect active HIV replication.[7] It should also be noted that decreased serum albumin and decreased cholesterol levels may be detected in advancing disease.[2–4,6]

■ Abnormalities in Hematological Studies

Clinically significant hematological abnormalities are common in HIV infection. These abnormalities can be caused by a single or, more likely, a number of factors in conjunction such as the direct effect of HIV infection, ineffective hematopoiesis, infiltrative disease, nutritional deficiencies, peripheral destruction secondary to splenomegaly or immune dysfunction or, perhaps most importantly, drug-induced hematological abnormalities.[6,8,9] Abnormalities are found in all stages of HIV infection and involve the bone marrow, cellular elements of the peripheral blood, and coagulation pathways.

The typical anemia, which is the direct effect of HIV infection, is normocytic and normochromic (Table 11–3). Microcytic anemia is fairly uncommon and should alert the clinician to the possibility of blood loss from Kaposi's sarcoma of the GI tract, lymphoma, or perhaps CMV coli-

TABLE 11–3. ANEMIA AND HIV

Causes of Normocytic Anemia:
HIV
Bone marrow infections
  Mycobacterium avium
  Mycobacterium tuberculosis
  Histoplasma capsulatum
  Coccidioides immitis
  Cryptococcus neoformans
  Pneumocystis carinii
  Leishmania donovani

Causes of Microcytic Anemia:
Kaposi's sarcoma of the GI tract
CMV colitis
Lymphoma

Causes of Macrocytic Anemia:
Zidovudine (AZT or Retrovir)
B-12 or folate deficiency secondary to malabsorption
Hemolytic anemia
Drugs: Dapsone or sulfa drugs

tis with resultant iron deficiency.[3] Since nutritional deficiency has been documented in HIV-infected individuals, folate, B_{12}, and iron studies may help in diagnosing the cause and treatment of the anemia.

Bone marrow abnormalities are common in HIV. In addition to the virus itself causing myelosuppression, infectious processes such as the atypical mycobacteria (*M. avium* and *M. kansasii*), histoplasmosis, cryptococcosis, and B19 parvovirus are known to aggravate or cause anemia.[8] Infectious causes of anemia should always be considered when the patient has unexplained constitutional symptoms, involvement of all blood cell lines, or a consistent decrease in hemoglobin without an alternative etiology.

Granulocytopenia is another commonly encountered cytopenia in HIV infection (Table 11–4). Like other cyto-

TABLE 11–4. CAUSES OF GRANULOCYTOPENIA

HIV
Infection
Malignancy
Drug-induced
  AZT (Retrovir)
  Trimethoprim-sulfamethoxazole (TMP-SMX)
  Amphotericin B
  Ganciclovir (DHPG)
  Acyclovir (Zovirax)
  Pyrimethamine
  IV Pentamidine
  Interferon
  Chemotherapy for Kaposi's sarcoma or lymphoma

penias, it may stem from HIV infection alone, be caused by a myelopathic process in the bone marrow, or more commonly be caused by drug therapy.[3,6] Only when the absolute granulocyte count falls below 750 does the risk of infection and sepsis become great.

Thrombocytopenia is the most frequent platelet abnormality associated with HIV infection. The etiology may be HIV related or may be a side effect of drug therapy. HIV-related immune thrombocytopenic purpura (ITP) is a diagnosis of exclusion and is properly diagnosed only when the patient has no other condition causing the thrombocytopenia.[10] HIV-related ITP may be associated with splenomegaly and is often found in conjunction with generalized lymphadenopathy. Common causes of drug-induced thrombocytopenia are TMP-SMX, amphotericin B, pyrimethamine, and ketoconazole. One unusual phenomenon is that AZT at higher doses than usual may actually increase the platelet count.

Prolonged activated partial thromboplastin times (PTT) are occasionally detected in patients with HIV infection. This is thought to be a result of "lupus-like" anticoagulants and is probably an acquired immunoglobulin that interferes with phospholipid-dependent coagulation, thus prolonging the PTT. Hemorrhagic tendencies have not been noted in these patients, and invasive procedures have been performed without an increased risk of bleeding.[4,6]

■ Abnormalities in Renal Function

Throughout the course of their illness, AIDS patients are at a high risk for renal complications. Systemic infection, sepsis, dehydration, hypoxia, and nephrotoxic drugs combine to decrease renal function and may permanently damage the kidneys.

Hyponatremia is one of the most common metabolic problems in patients with HIV infection. Gastrointestinal salt losses from diarrhea and free water repletion are the most common cause of hyponatremia. Volume repletion with normal saline generally corrects this condition.[3] Another cause of hyponatremia is the syndrome of inappropriate antidiuretic hormone secretion (SIADH). Syndrome of inappropriate antidiuretic hormone secretion is most often caused by infection or mass lesions in the brain or lung of AIDS patients. Additionally, SIADH is associated with euvolemic hyponatremia and is primarily managed by fluid restriction.

There are numerous etiologies for lesions in the kidneys of AIDS patients that cause clinical evidence of renal disease. One of these lesions is focal segmental glomerulosclerosis.[3,4,6] Focal segmental glomerulosclerosis primarily occurs among IV drug users and in black males. It still remains controversial whether this is an HIV- or IDU-related event. However, the most significant factor contributing to kidney failure is nephrotoxic drugs used in therapy for opportunistic infections (Table 11–5).

TABLE 11–5. NEPHROTOXIC DRUGS

Amphotericin B*
Pentamidine
Foscarnet*
Ganciclovir (DHPG)
Sulfa drugs
Aminoglycosides*
Acyclovir (Zovirax)
Rifampin
Flucytosine
Nonsteroidal antiinflammatory drugs

*May also be associated with magnesium-wasting nephropathy.

■ Abnormalities in Liver Function

Abnormalities in liver function commonly occur in HIV and AIDS patients. Liver dysfunction may be related to preexisting hepatic disease, ethanol usage, infections, neoplasms, or drug toxicity. Three distinct clinical syndromes have been recognized: (1) diffuse hepatocellular injury, (2) granulomatous hepatitis, and (3) sclerosing cholangitis.[3,4,6] Abnormal liver function tests are frequently a result of fatty infiltration of the liver or other nonspecific changes.

Diffuse hepatitis is most commonly the result of drug toxicity. Less frequently, hepatitis C or chronic active hepatitis B causes diffuse disease. The clinical picture of diffuse hepatocellular disease shows low-grade fever, hepatomegaly, jaundice, and, in severe cases, ascites. Rapidly rising SGPT (ALT), SGOT (AST), and elevated bilirubin levels are common.[2,3,6]

Granulomatous hepatitis is associated with mycobacterial or fungal disease as well as drug toxicity. This produces an obstructive or cholestatic enzyme pattern. Other infective processes that have been noted to affect the liver are CMV and cryptosporidiosis. Fever and constitutional symptoms are prominent in infectious processes.[4,6] Liver function tests demonstrate progressively rising levels of alkaline phosphatase, SGOT, and SGPT. Bilirubin concentrations are less often affected.[2,4,6]

Sclerosing cholangitis has been recognized in AIDS patients. The etiologies and pathophysiology are not known. Patients present with nonspecific abdominal complaints and progressive cholestasis. Retrograde endoscopy has demonstrated single and multiple areas of narrowing or dilation of intrahepatic and extrahepatic ducts.[3] In long-term cases, progressive jaundice and liver failure develop.

Hepatotoxic medications should be withheld when the patient has clinical symptoms of hepatitis. Often the liver enzymes may be elevated as much as fourfold without any clinical signs of hepatitis. Some of the more common hepatotoxic medications are the antituberculars (rifampin, pyrazinamide, and isoniazid) and the antifungals (fluconazole, ketoconazole, and itraconazole); an infrequently toxic drug is TMP-SMX.

■ Abnormalities in Pancreatic Function

Pancreatic disease in AIDS patients has received little attention until recently.[3] The most common causes of elevated lipase levels, but not necessarily pancreatic disease, are the antiretrovirals, didanosine (ddI) and zalcitabine (ddC). Intravenous pentamidine therapy for *Pneumocystis* pneumonia has been associated with hypoglycemia because of selective damage to beta cells in the islets of Langerhans.[3,4,6] If this injury is sufficiently severe or prolonged, hyperglycemia and insulin-dependent diabetes can result. Pentamidine may also cause overt pancreatitis. The combination of zalcitibine and pentamidine should be avoided. Patients with a significant history of alcohol use should be given didanosine with careful monitoring.

Lipase is a more specific marker of pancreatic function; however, in acute pancreatitis, the amylase level may rise more rapidly initially but typically returns to normal range more quickly than lipase.[2,3] An elevation in lipase and/or amylase, without clinical or symptoms signs of pancreatitis, does not necessitate discontinuation of didanosine or zalcitibine.

Systemic complications of Kaposi's sarcoma are known to affect the pancreas. Systemic CMV, MAI, and fungal infections may also injure the pancreas, although pancreatic involvement is rarely noticed until autopsy.[3,4,6]

References

1. Ravel R. *Clinical Laboratory Medicine.* Chicago: Year Book Medical Publishers; 1989.
2. Fischbach F. *A Manual of Laboratory and Diagnostic Tests.* Philadelphia: JB Lippincott; 1992.
3. Masci J. *Primary and Ambulatory Care of the HIV Infected Adult.* St. Louis, MO: Mosby; 1992.
4. Joshi V, ed. *Pathology of AIDS and Other Manifestations of HIV Infection.* New York: Igaku-Shoin; 1990.
5. Jewell M, Swee D. Asymptomatic HIV infection a primary care disease. *Postgrad Med.* 1992; 92(5):155–166.
6. Sande M, Volberding P. *The Medical Management of AIDS.* Philadelphia: WB Saunders Co; 1990.
7. Polis MA, Masur H. Predicting the progression to AIDS. *Am J Med.* 1990;89:701–704.
8. Mir N, Costello C, Luckit J, et al. HIV disease and bone marrow changes: A study of sixty cases. *Eur J Haematol.* 1989;42(4):339–343.
9. Mitsuyasu R, Lambertus M, Goetz MB. Transfusion dependent anemia in a patient with AIDS. *Clin Infect Dis.* 1992;15:533–539.
10. Ratner L. HIV associated autoimmune thrombocytopenia purpura: a review, *Am J Med.* 1989;86:194–198.

Chapter Twelve

DERMATOLOGIC MANIFESTATIONS

SANDEE W. ROQUEMORE, PA-C
ANGELA WEGMANN, PA-C
SALAH AYACHI, PhD, PA-C

The skin is a commonly affected organ in patients who are HIV positive. Some dermatologic diseases, such as shingles, can serve as markers of underlying HIV infection, and others, such as an epidemic form of Kaposi's sarcoma, are diagnostic of AIDS.

Most skin disorders found in immunosuppressed patients can also be seen in immunocompetent hosts. In the HIV-infected immunosuppressed individual, these diseases are more extensive and refractory to treatment. Skin lesions that are most common in HIV patients can be divided into three broad categories: infectious, noninfectious, and neoplastic.

■ Infectious

Viral Infections

Varicella Zoster Virus (Shingles, VZV). Clinical zoster occurs as a reactivation of varicella zoster virus and is seen with increased frequency in immunosuppressed patients. Zoster occurs commonly in the elderly but very infrequently in those under 35 years of age. Clinicians should be alerted to looking for underlying HIV disease in any young patient who presents with zoster.

Zoster occurs only in patients who have previously been infected with VZV ("chickenpox"). Upon resolution of the chickenpox, the virus travels from the cutaneous lesions to the sensory neurons and into the dorsal root ganglia where it remains dormant. In the normal host it takes years for the virus to reactivate, at which time the patient develops shingles. As with most diseases, the clinical course may vary. However, most patients experience a prodrome of sensory disturbances in the distribution of the involved dermatome prior to appearance of the lesions. The patient may report burning, tingling, or pain and tenderness to palpation in the affected area followed by appearance of the lesions 3 to 5 days later.

The lesions most often begin as papules and evolve into vesicles with an erythematous base. The vesicles may evolve into multiple small pustules that later begin to crust and then resolve. New lesions may appear for another 5 to 7 days. Oral acyclovir (Zovirax) at 800 mg five times daily for 10 days is the therapy of choice. Occasionally patients may require a more prolonged course of treatment.

Herpes zoster may involve a single dermatome or multiple dermatomes and can be recurrent or disseminated. Unidermatomal zoster is the most common and is easy to define. The lesions involve one dermatome and do not cross the midline. Multidermatomal zoster involves two or more dermatomes. Recurrent zoster is diagnosed in patients with multiple bouts of shingles. In disseminated zoster, 20 or more lesions are found in widely scattered areas from the primary dermatomes. Occasionally patients will develop disseminated disease with visceral involvement, especially of the lungs and CNS. Visceral involvement without cutaneous dissemination occurs very rarely.

Both postherpetic neuralgia and scarring from shingles are more common in HIV-positive than in immunocompetent patients.[1] Some experts feel that postherpetic neuralgia may last for weeks to months and can effectively be treated with the tricyclic antidepressants (amitriptyline or imipramine) or antiepileptics (phenytoin or tegretol).

Herpes Simplex Virus (HSV). With increasing immunosuppression, HSV recurrences can be progressive and persistent. Active lesions in this population are typically reactivation of latent infection. Acyclovir-resistant strains complicate the picture by confusing the diagnosis and occasionally presenting with atypical features.

The acute vesicular eruption rapidly evolves into chronic nonhealing ulcerations. The most common sites of infection are perianal, genital, and orofacial in order of frequency. Erosions at the usual sites can enlarge and deepen and, if left untreated, can coalesce into lesions up to 20 cm in diameter.[2] Lesions may also extend from the oropharynx to the esophagus, causing severe odynophagia. Secondary bacterial infections, particularly of perianal ulcers, occur commonly and may mask the original process. Oral acyclovir, 200 mg every 4 hours while awake, is the preferred therapy. Oral antibiotics should be added to this regimen if secondary infection is suspected. Severe disease may require IV acyclovir at 5 to 10 mg/kg every 8 hours for 14 days followed by the oral regimen. Failure to respond necessitates immediate evaluation for acyclovir-resistant strains.

Molluscum Contagiosum. This is a cutaneous pox virus infection that, in immunocompetent patients, is usually sexually transmitted and self-limiting. However, in the HIV-positive patient the clinical course differs significantly. It remains unknown whether the lesions represent de novo infection or reactivated latent infections. However, its predilection for trunk and face, along with its occurrence in advanced symptomatic HIV disease, favors the latter. The incidence approximates 10% to 20%.[2]

Molluscum appears as flesh-colored umbilicated papules, 1 to 3 mm in diameter, distributed usually to face, neck, scalp, and trunk. Atypical lesions growing up to 10 mm will commonly occur in this patient population. Diagnosis is usually made clinically, but early biopsy is recommended for atypical lesions. Lesions that may be confused with molluscum include cutaneous cryptococcosis, histoplasmosis, coccidioidomycosis, verruca, and squamous cell carcinoma. Treatment modalities include liquid nitrogen, electrocoagulation, and curettage. Retin-A cream, 0.01%, applied once daily may suppress new lesions. In most instances a cure is not accomplished.

Human Papilloma Virus (HPV). Human papilloma virus infections such as verrucae vulgare (common warts) and condylomata (anogenital warts) are common in HIV-infected patients. They occur in the same physical distribution as in HIV-negative patients but are more numerous and refractory to treatment.

Verrucae vulgare of the hands are extremely common. It is also typical for the lesions to coalesce into large plaque-like areas. Flat warts of the beard and plantar surfaces are also frequently seen. Treatment is difficult, and recurrence is the norm. Management options for these lesions include cryotherapy, keratolytics, electrodesiccation, and laser therapy.

Condylomata, which occur as flesh-colored warts, are sexually transmitted and can be found on the skin, oropharynx, genitalia, and/or anal area. The lesions may not become apparent for weeks to years after the patient has been infected with HPV. They normally first appear as flesh-colored, pink, or red papules and may develop into the common "cauliflower-like" mass for which it is so well known. Condyloma treatment options include cryo-surgery, laser surgery, electrocautery, and podophyllin; patients are usually referred to the dermatologist. In-tralesional interferon is also being used in clinical trials. Even after appropriate treatment, condyloma recurs in a large number of patients. It is important to keep in mind that squamous cell carcinoma may also present as rapidly growing genital vegetative lesions near the vulva and/or anus.[3]

Fungal Infections

Candida. Candidiasis can present as a cutaneous, perianal, or vaginal infection. The lesions usually appear as erythem-atous tender patches in the groin, axillary, or inframammary areas with satellite papules in the periphery. In the male, *Candida* can produce balanitis and distal urethritis. In fe-males, vaginal candidiasis is common and can be recurrent and extremely bothersome. *Candida* can also produce acute or chronic paronychia. Treatment of *Candida* infections in-cludes drying of wet areas and application of antifungal powders (nystatin) and creams (clotrimazole). If topical agents fail to clear the infection, oral fluconazole, 100 to 200 mg orally every day for at least 14 days, may be used. Oral agents such as griseofulvin, 500 mg every day for at least 6 months, are usually needed to treat onychomycosis and paronychial infections.

Tinea. Dermatophytid tinea infections are quite common in the HIV-infected host and present the same as in their HIV-negative counterpart. Tinea pedis ("athlete's foot") is seen most often, and it presents with the usual maceration of the interdigital areas with scaling of the foot. Onychomycosis is commonly seen in conjunction with tinea pedis.

Tinea cruris ("jock itch") is also common in HIV-infected hosts. Typically it presents as erythematous, scaly, pruriginous plaques with sharply demarcated borders. It appears in the genitocrural folds and may extend to the inner thighs and scrotum. If the patient is severely immunosuppressed, the erythema may not be present, and the lesions may not have the area of central clearing that is so typical of tinea cruris.[3]

Tinea corporis ("ringworm") usually first appears as scaly annular plaque-like lesions with central clearing. Like tinea cruris, tinea corporis may look atypical if the patient is severely immunosuppressed. In this instance, borders of the lesions may not be elevated, and the central clearing may not be present.[3]

Normal treatment modalities can be used in attempts to eradicate these fungal infections. Topical antifungal creams (ie, naftifine 1% twice daily) can be used to treat tinea pedis and tinea cruris; however, for tinea corporis, a systemic antifungal such as fluconazole, 50 mg orally every day for 1 month may need to be added.[3]

Systemic Fungal Infections. Several systemic fungal infections can manifest as cutaneous lesions. Cryptococcosis occurs in approximately 10% of all patients with AIDS. Most of the cases involve the CNS, but the skin may also be involved with lesions much like those of molluscum contagiosum. They appear as umbilicated, white papules or occasionally as papules with a central area of crusting. These lesions are found most often on the face and usually occur in groups. Cutaneous cryptococcosis is always associated with systemic infection. Patients with cryptococcosis are hospitalized and treated with amphotericin B followed by fluconazole for maintenance therapy (see Chapter 7).[3]

Histoplasmosis is another common fungal infection that presents with cutaneous lesions in about 10% of patients with disseminated histoplasmosis. Lesions secondary to histoplasmosis can present as papules, papulonecrotic lesions, cup-shaped papules, vegetative plaques, or diffuse purpura-like lesions.[3] Histoplasmosis is also treated with amphotericin B, followed by itraconazole for maintenance (see Chapter 7).

■ Noninfectious

Seborrheic Dermatitis (SD). This is an "exaggerated dandruff" condition that affects those areas of greatest sebaceous activity (nasolabial folds, eyebrows, and mustache). In patients with AIDS, the incidence of SD has been estimated at 40% to 80%, whereas in HIV-seropositive patients the incidence is 20% to 40%, as compared to only 3% to 5% in those who are immunocompetent.[4] Seborrheic dermatitis manifests with greasy scales. The etiology is thought to be multifactorial and partly related to overgrowth of several different cutaneous fungi.

Generally, treatment consists of 1% hydrocortisone cream applied to the affected areas two or three times a day. Since SD is thought to have a fungal component, many are beginning to use a combination of hydrocortisone and antifungal cream. It must be stressed that treatment for SD is not curative, only palliative. Once treatment is stopped, the lesions will recur.

Psoriasis. Psoriasis is a papulosquamous dermatosis that is also associated with HIV infection. As with most other dermatoses, psoriasis presents with pronounced severity. New onset of explosive psoriasis or sudden exacerbations in an individual with previous chronic stable psoriasis is the usual picture and can be a marker of undiagnosed

HIV infection. In the immunocompetent patient, psoriasis is usually a mild disease limited to extensor surfaces and affects 1% to 2% of the general population.[5]

Psoriatic lesions in HIV-positive patients are identical to those seen in the general public, although the clinical disease differs in that several subsets of lesions may be found in the same patient. Patients may have papules (guttate), pustules, plaques, extensive exfoliative erythroderma, or some combination of these. Typical nail changes are seen ranging from pitting to severe destruction.

Treatment is complicated in that most treatments, including ultraviolet B (UVB), involve some degree of immunosuppression. Care must be taken to use the lowest effective dosages. Therapeutic modalities include emollients, salicylic acid ointment, topical corticosteroids, crude coal tar, ultraviolet light, and etretinate.

Zidovudine at high doses (200 mg four times a day) has been used for prompt symptomatic relief of pruritus and clearing of lesions in 6 to 8 weeks. Methotrexate is contraindicated as it has been associated with rapid immunosuppression and death.[5]

Eosinophilic Pustular Folliculitis (EPF). Eosinophilic pustular folliculitis, also commonly called HIV-associated eosinophilic folliculitis, is a chronic and extremely pruritic eruption that is clinically similar to bacterial folliculitis. Lesions begin as small papules or pustules that typically involve the face, neck, trunk, or extremities. It is common for patients with EPF to present with lichenified or even ulcerated areas secondary to intense scratching of the lesions. The exact etiology of EPF is unknown, but histopathologic findings include innumerable eosinophils within the fundibula of hair follicles.[6] Occasionally, the follicles may rupture, resulting in perifolliculitis.

Treatment of EPF is difficult. Oral antihistamines can be used to alleviate some of the pruritus. Ultraviolet B phototherapy is the treatment of choice but should be undertaken with caution because of the possibility of reactivation of latent HIV infection and reduction of the T4 cell population. In many instances, once the phototherapy is discontinued, the symptoms will reappear.

Pruritic Papular Eruption (PPE) of HIV. This is a poorly defined chronic pruritus and dermatitis seen frequently (up to about 80% incidence) in HIV-positive patients. The etiology of this eruption and the accompanying pruritus is unknown.

The eruption consists of symmetrical, flesh-colored to erythematous, papules involving the trunk, neck, and extremities to varying degrees. Numerous secondary changes including multiple excoriations, postinflammatory hyperpigmentation, and prurigo-like nodules are typically seen. The eruption may not be follicular and does not coalesce to form plaques. The course usually waxes and wanes over periods of 1 to 24 months.

Typical histological features include superficial and middermal perivascular and perifollicular lymphocytic infiltrates with variable numbers of eosinophils. Other common conditions that can be mistaken for PPE include eosinophilic folliculitis and drug eruption.

Treatment includes UVB treatments thrice weekly, topical corticosteroids, emollients, and antihistamines. Results are variable; the pruritus is usually refractory to most standard oral and topical treatments.[7] Spontaneous resolution can occur at any time during the clinical course.

Xerosis. Severe xerosis is extremely common in HIV-infected hosts, and several different reasons for the changes in the skin have been postulated. A few of these include reduced production of sebum and exocrine sweat, epidermal cell kinetic abnormality, poor nutrition or poor absorption of nutrients, or a combination of these factors. Treatment modalities include frequent application of emollients, proper nutrition, and avoidance of drying soaps.

Hair Changes. Multiple nonspecific hair changes have also been observed in HIV patients. These may include alopecia, loss of luster, and straightening of previously curly hair. These are felt to be secondary to a combination of HIV infection of the follicular epithelium and nutritional abnormalities. Many patients also experience elongation of eyelashes because of prolonged anlagen phase of growth, a phenomenon called trichomegaly.[8]

Drug Eruptions. Drug-related eruptions are quite common in HIV-infected patients. The rash usually consists of pruritic pink to red macules or papules and may last for several weeks to months after discontinuation of the offending drug. The most common agent that causes a drug eruption is trimethoprim-sulfamethoxazole. Others include clindamycin, cephalexin, and rifabutin. Treatment for drug eruption normally consists of cessation of the offending drug and antihistamines as needed.

Scabies. This is a condition caused by a mite (arthropod) that is spread by skin-to-skin contact as a result of overcrowding, poverty, or sexual activity. The presence of a mite, its eggs, and its waste products causes an allergic response characterized by severe intractable pruritus. Characteristic lesions are "burrows," brownish erythematous papules, and vesicles.

Sites of predilection are the hands, interdigital webs, flexor wrists, nipples, axilla, buttocks, penis, and feet. Diagnosis is established by scraping of burrows or papules and microscopic examination to reveal the eggs or parts of the body of the mite. Norwegian ("crusted") scabies is also seen in immunosuppressed hosts as crusted plaques and marked hyperkeratosis at the usual sites.

Treatment is with 1% lindane lotion or 10% crotamiton cream.

■ Neoplastic

Kaposi's Sarcoma

Kaposi's sarcoma (KS) is a multifocal neoplasm that can affect any organ in the body. Skin is the most commonly involved organ, and it can present in a variety of forms, colors, shapes, and distribution patterns. Kaposi's sarcoma is the only opportunistic disease than can occur in the setting of normal T4 counts. Histologically, KS lesions consist of small vascular spaces, multiple abnormal lymphocytes, spindle-like cells, blood vessels, and extravasated red cells.[9]

Many researchers have sought an infectious agent in the pathogenesis of KS. CMV has been thoroughly researched, and it currently seems unlikely that it is the culprit. Some feel that herpes viruses may indirectly affect the development of KS through the activation of leukocytes and induction of soluble factors.[9] Studies are still under way to pinpoint an exact infectious agent.

Kaposi's sarcoma skin lesions normally begin as tiny macular violaceous areas. The lesion may enlarge and possibly become elevated to form a plaque-like lesion. The plaques sometimes enlarge further into nodules. These lesions are typically nonpruritic, painless, and may have some surrounding edema, which is felt to be secondary to lymphatic obstruction. Although KS lesions are painless, it is possible for them to become ulcerated and thereby cause local pain. Suspicious lesions should always be biopsied. Mucous membrane, gastrointestinal, and pulmonary involvement, ranging from involvement of the oral cavity, stomach, colon, small intestine, large bowel, and lungs, may be found in advanced cases.

Treatment options include observation, excision, radiation, and chemotherapy. Excision is only reasonable for small lesions one wishes to remove for cosmetic purposes. Radiation is also used primarily for smaller lesions because complete resolution of larger lesions with radiation is rare. Chemotherapy is normally reserved for patients with rapidly progressing lesions or patients with visceral involvement. Alpha interferon is effective in controlling KS in patients with high T4 levels. Multiple agents have been studied, including bleomycin, vincristine, vinblastine, and adriamycin, among others, all with varying degrees of success. Even with a good response to chemotherapy, KS will usually relapse quickly after the therapy has been stopped.

References

1. Cockerell CJ. Cutaneous and histologic signs of HIV infection other than Kaposi's sarcoma. In: Wormser GP, ed. *AIDS and Other Manifestations of HIV Infection.* New York: Raven Press; 1992:465.

2. Dover JS, Johnson RA. Cutaneous manifestations of human immunodeficiency virus infection, part I. *Arch Dermatol.* 1991;127:1383–1391.

3. Berger TG, Greene I. Bacterial, viral, fungal, and parasitic infections in HIV disease and AIDS. In: James W, ed. *AIDS: A Ten-Year Perspective.* Philadelphia: WB Saunders; 1991:478–485.

4. Mathes BM, Douglas MC. Seborrheic dermatitis in patients with AIDS. *J Am Acad Dermatol.* 1985;13:947–951.

5. Sadick N, NcNutt NS, Kaplan M. Papulosquamous dermatoses of AIDS. *J Am Acad Dermatol.* 1990;22:1270–1277.

6. Cockerell CJ, Cutaneous and histologic signs of HIV infection other than Kaposi's sarcoma. In: Wormser

GP, ed. *AIDS and Other Manifestations of HIV Infection.* New York: Raven Press; 1992:473.

7. Pardo RJ, Bogaert MA, Penneys NS, et al. UVB phototherapy of the pruritic papular eruption of the acquired immunodeficiency syndrome. *J Am Acad Dermatol.* 1992; 26:423–428.

8. Cockerell CJ. Non infectious inflammatory skin diseases in HIV infected individuals. In: James W, ed. *AIDS: A Ten-Year Perspective.* Philadelphia: WB Saunders; 1991:537.

9. Levine AM, Gill PS, Salahuddin SZ. Neoplastic complications of HIV infection. In: Wormser GP, ed. *AIDS and Other Manifestations of HIV Infection.* New York: Raven Press; 1992:444.

Chapter Thirteen

....
....
....
....

WOMEN AND HIV

TERESA NEWMAN, PA-C
MARK G. MARTENS, MD

■ The Epidemiology of AIDS in Women

The first female case of AIDS in the United States was reported in 1981.[1] Women are one of the fastest growing groups infected with the AIDS virus. Women constituted 9% of the first 100,000 persons with AIDS as compared to 12% in the second 100,000 persons.[2] Also, the CDC reports that the first 100,000 cases were reported during an eight-year period, while the second 100,000 cases were reported in only a two-year period.[2] AIDS is the leading cause of death among women aged 25 to 34 years in New York City.[1]

According to the CDC, the sources of HIV infection in women are approximately ranked as follows: IV drug use, 51%; heterosexual activity, 34%; blood transfusion, 8%; and unknown, 7%.[2] Approximately 85% of the women with AIDS are of childbearing potential, 15 to 44 years of age.[3] Therefore, there is the risk of transmission of HIV to a child during pregnancy, delivery, and breast-feeding.

■ Diagnosis

Historically, women have not been diagnosed until they were further along in the course of AIDS.[1] Factors contributing to this late diagnosis may include poor access to health care, poor utilization of health care, and the low degree of suspicion of HIV-related disease by health care providers of women. Also, the women at high risk may not be aware of the early symptoms of HIV.

Gynecologic symptoms are often the first sign of the HIV infection in women.[4] However, these infections were not included in the previous CDC criteria, and clinicians may not suspect HIV infection. Gynecologic symptoms included in the 1993 revised classification system for HIV infection are vulvovaginal candidiasis that is persistent, frequent, or poorly responsive to therapy; cervical dysplasia from moderate to invasive; pelvic inflammatory disease, especially those with tubo-ovarian abscess; and herpes simplex ulcer lasting more than 1 month.[5] Other gynecologic symptoms that are not included are genital ulcers, human papilloma virus, syphilis, and condyloma acuminata.[4] These will be discussed in more detail under Medical Complications in this chapter.

■ HIV Testing in Women

The Centers for Disease Control and Prevention recommends that all women of childbearing age with high-risk behaviors should be counseled and tested for HIV.[6] Ulcers are a port of entry for the AIDS virus and other sexually transmitted diseases.[1] Therefore, anyone with an ulcerative lesion on the genitalia should be counseled and tested for HIV.

■ Initial Work-up for Women with HIV

The work-up mentioned later in this book (see Chapter 14) needs to be performed. However, there are additional components in women that need to be evaluated when HIV is detected.[7]

1. Thorough gynecologic history including menstrual, obstetric, contraceptive, and sexual histories.
2. Physical examination including breast and pelvic exam.
3. Labs: Pap smear, cervical cultures for *Chlamydia* and gonorrhea, VDRL, and pregnancy test (if indicated).
4. Mammogram for women between 35 and 39 years, every other year for women through 49 years, and every year 50 years and older.
5. Colposcopy (optional, but highly suggested in light of new data).

■ Medical Complications in Women with HIV Infection

Candida esophagitis and *Pneumocystis carinii* pneumonia are the most frequent AIDS-defining events in women with HIV.[1] However, there are several gynecologic manifestations in the HIV-infected woman.

Human Papillomavirus and Cervical Disease

Human papillomavirus (HPV) is one of the most common sexually transmitted diseases in the United States.[1] HPV may present as anogenital warts (condyloma acuminata), as cervical dysplasia, or as invasive carcinoma of the cervix on Pap smear. HIV-infected women have a high prevalence of HPV and abnormal Pap smears.[1] Therefore, it is important that an adequate Pap smear is done at least once a year in

HIV-infected women. If the Pap smear is inadequate or abnormal, colposcopy should be performed.[7]

Herpes Simplex Virus

Genital herpes, or herpes simplex virus, may present suddenly in an HIV-infected woman and become persistent, widespread, and more painful than HSV in a non-HIV-infected woman.[1,4] Treatment is not different from the treatment stated in Chapter 12. As with other immuno-compromised diseases, HIV-infected women with HSV lesions may shed HIV more frequently than noninfected women and increase the risk of HIV transmission to their sexual partners.

Chancroid

Although this sexually transmitted disease was once rarely seen in the United States, its prevalence has been increasing in the past decade.[4] Chancroid presents as an acute painful ulcer on the external genitalia with inguinal lymphadenopathy.

Treatment is usually effective with a single dose of a quinolone or ceftriaxone. If this fails, a 3-day regimen of a fluoroquinolone (eg, ciprofloxacin hydrochloride) should be considered.[7] The incidence of treatment failure in women is increased in those with HIV.

Syphilis

In HIV-infected individuals, syphilis appears to take a more aggressive course and progresses quickly from primary to tertiary syphilis.[4] Treatment of primary, secondary, and tertiary syphilis in the HIV-infected patient, regardless of pregnancy, should be with benzathine penicillin IM once a week for three consecutive weeks.[8] Follow-up with serial tests such as VDRL and RPR should be done at 1, 2, 3, 6, 9, and 12 months.[1] If the test fails to decrease fourfold or continue to rise within 6 months, the HIV-infected woman should have her cerebrospinal fluid tested by VDRL and be retreated as outlined above.

Studies suggest that a history of syphilis is a high-risk factor for HIV infection.[1,4] Therefore, HIV counseling and testing should be offered to women who are being treated for syphilis. Likewise, women with HIV should also be tested for syphilis, since the prevalence of syphilis is also on the rise in the United States.

HIV Genital Ulcers

Besides the ulcers that occur with chancroid, syphilis, and herpes simplex virus, a new entity, HIV genital ulcer, has recently been described in a few women with HIV.[7] This type of ulcer was cultured for herpes simplex virus and chancroid, and dark-field microscopy was performed. Although all test results were negative, the patient was treated for HSV, chancroid, and syphilis with no resolution of the ulcer. A trial of zidovudine (AZT) was started, and the ulcer rapidly healed. Primary HIV ulcer should be in the differential of HIV-infected women with genital ulcers. However, these ulcers may appear on other parts of the body where there are mucous membranes.

Pelvic Inflammatory Disease

Although the infecting organisms, gonorrhea, *Chlamydia*, and aerobic and anaerobic species, are the same in both HIV-infected and noninfected women, HIV-infected women do not have classic presentation of their infection. Abscesses are seen more frequently, and surgical intervention occurs more often in HIV-infected women.[7] Leukocytosis with pelvic inflammatory disease (PID) is seen less frequently in HIV-infected women.

Inpatient treatment of PID in HIV-infected women could be justified since they are immunocompromised.

Cefoxitin, 2 g IV every 6 hours plus doxycycline, 100 mg every 12 hours orally or IV, is one of several regimens that should be continued for at least 48 hours after the patient clinically improves. Doxycycline, 100 mg orally two times a day for a total of 10 to 14 days, is recommended after discharge from the hospital. Symptoms that persist despite this treatment may be a sign of a failing immune system.

Vaginal Candidiasis

Although vaginal candidiasis is a common gynecologic infection in all women, recurrent vaginal candidiasis occurs more often in those with HIV.[4,7] Therefore, recurrent vaginal candidiasis, as in five to six infections in a year, may be an early warning sign of HIV infection.[1]

Treatment for the initial episode of vaginal candidiasis in the HIV-infected woman should be the standard topical antifungal medication such as clotrimazole. In the absence of correctable causes (ie, oral contraceptive or antibiotics), recurrent or resistant vaginal candidiasis is treated orally with ketoconazole, 400 mg a day for 14 days followed by 5-day courses each month for 6 months.[7] Liver functions should be monitored carefully with treatment. Fluconazole oral therapy is currently under review by the FDA for the treatment of vaginal candidiasis and may be a suitable alternative in the future.

Pregnancy

Many women learn of their HIV status from prenatal screening.[7] At this point, it is ideal to counsel the patient on either pregnancy termination or continuation. The rate of vertical transmission, from mother to fetus, is 25% to 35%.[9] Other studies have shown broader ranges.

Women may acquire their first assessment and HIV care during pregnancy (Table 13–1).[7] The usual approach to the asymptomatic infected individual need

TABLE 13–1. EVALUATION OF PREGNANT HIV-INFECTED WOMEN. THE UNIVERSITY OF TEXAS MEDICAL BRANCH, GALVESTON, TEXAS

Prenatal

Initial visit

    Antibodies to toxoplasma and cytomegalovirus.

    Tuberculosis skin testing (Mantoux)

    Cervical cultures for *Neisseria gonorrhoeae* and *Chlamydia trachomatis*

    Hepatitis B surface antigen

    VDRL

    Cryptococcal antigen

    Beta-2 microglobulin

    SMA12

T4 lymphocytes every 3 months (monthly if < 300 mm^3)

Administer Pneumovax vaccine

Delivery

Urine or cervical culture for cytomegalovirus

Repeat toxoplasma titers for seronegative patients

Prenatal and Postpartum Therapy

If T4 < 500 mm^3, discuss zidovudine (AZT) therapy

If T4 < 200 mm^3, encourage PCP prophylaxis and AZT

not be altered. CD4 counts should be checked every 3 months to determine if she should begin zidovudine, or *Pneumocystis carinii* pneumonia (PCP) prophylactic treatment. Treatment of the pregnant woman should not be different from the nonpregnant woman. There are very few, if any, therapies that have caused sufficient fetal risks that would justify treatment modification at this time.

PCP prophylaxis should not be withheld from a pregnant woman with a T4 count less than 200 mm^3.[7,9] PCP has been associated with low T4 counts just as in nonpregnant women. Sulfamethoxazole or aerosolized pentamidine could be used. Fetal and neonatal bilirubin toxicity with sulfamethoxazole should be of concern. Kernicterus has been found with the use of sulfamethoxazole in premature infants. Therefore, sulfamethoxazole may be used in the first and second trimesters, and aerosolized pentamidine during the third trimester. Aerosolized pentamidine has low serum levels and limits fetal exposure.

The use of zidovudine should be offered to pregnant women with a T4 count less than 500 mm^3, preferably beyond the first trimester after the risks and benefits have been discussed.[7,9] These include anemia, nausea, vomiting, possibly fetal malformations, and improved immune status.

■ Management at Delivery and Postpartum

Universal precautions should be used on every patient, not limited to HIV-infected women. Protective eyewear should be worn during speculum examination for rupture of membranes and during delivery. The traditional mouth-operated DeLee's suction catheter should not be used to suction meconium from the newborn's respiratory tract.[9] Instead, the suction catheter can be attached to wall suction with long tubing.

Since the rate of vertical or placental transmission is approximately 25% to 35%, all fetuses should be treated as uninfected while in labor.[9] Precautions should be used to prevent horizontal transmission, or transmission from the mother to the infant. The mother may be allowed to handle her infant, but care should be taken to prevent exposure to maternal secretions. HIV has been isolated in breast milk.[8] The American College of Obstetricians and Gynecologists has recommended that HIV-infected women not breast feed.

■ Family Planning

HIV-infected women still have the right to choose their contraceptive method.[10] Having HIV does not seem to deter some women from becoming pregnant. Many women feel that they are leaving a legacy and have a bond to their partner through the child. There are, however, many HIV-infected women who do not want to become pregnant. These women need to be counseled on the different types of contraception, along with their advantages and disadvantages.

Surgical sterilization should not be encouraged or discouraged.[7] If chosen, as a contraceptive option, it may be performed in the standard manner.

Barrier methods such as condoms may protect against HIV and sexually transmitted diseases but do not have the efficacy rates that other contraceptives such as oral contraceptives and Norplant have in preventing pregnancy. Other barrier methods such as the diaphragm and the sponge are not as effective as a contraceptive or as protection from HIV or sexually transmitted diseases.

Oral contraceptives and the longer-acting hormonal contraceptives such as Norplant and Depo-Provera are not contraindicated in HIV-infected women at this time.[7] Studies are ongoing to see if the hormones in these contraceptives alter the natural course of HIV.

The intrauterine device (IUD) should be discouraged in women with HIV because of the increased susceptibility to ascending infections that could lead to pelvic inflammatory disease. Women with IUDs tend to have an increased amount of bleeding, which could transmit HIV more readily.

If the HIV-infected woman chooses a contraceptive other than condoms, she must be reminded to use condoms to protect her partner from HIV and herself from sexually transmitted diseases.

■ Psychosocial Aspects of HIV in Women

Women are usually the caregivers of the HIV-infected families.[7] The woman may not access health care because of her need to provide care for her children and/or partner. A woman may also encounter discrimination when going for drug rehabilitation, HIV therapeutics, and research trials because she is pregnant or is of childbearing age.

For substance abusers, there is incentive to change their drug habits while being pregnant.[10] This is a time in their life when they feel better about themselves and are responsible for another life.

With African-Americans and Hispanics, the woman may be physically abused if she suggests condom use to her partner.[10] Some Hispanic men feel that condoms are to be used only with women of loose moral character and not with their wife or steady partner. A lack of trust may develop between partners when concerns over AIDS are verbalized.

Women are less likely than men to question their partner about sexual preferences or drug habits.[10] When questioning occurs, there is no guarantee that the partner will tell the truth.

■ Summary

Since women have comprised a small number of cases of HIV infection, useful clinical information on the epidemiology, detection, and treatment of HIV has just begun to be elucidated. Studies have supported the recent change in the CDC Surveillance AIDS case definition and classification to include the predominant diseases of women. Additional studies will contribute much more to this area of patient care.

References

1. Allen MH. Primary care of women infected with the human immunodeficiency virus. *Obstet Gynecol Clin North Am.* 1990;17:557–569.

2. Centers for Disease Control. The second 100,000 cases of acquired immunodeficiency syndrome—United States, June, 1981–December, 1991. *MMWR.* 1992;41: 28–29.

3. Ellerbrock TV, Rogers MF. Epidemiology of human immunodeficiency virus infection in women in the United States. *Obstet Gynecol Clin North Am.* 1990;17: 523–544.

4. Smeltzer VT, Whipple B. Women and HIV infection. *Image J Nurs Sch.* 1991;23:249–255.

5. Centers for Disease Control. 1993 revised classification system for HIV infection and expanded surveillance case definition for AIDS among adolescents and adults. *MMWR.* 1992;41(RR-17):1–19.

6. Centers for Disease Control. Public health service guidelines for counseling and antibody testing to prevent HIV infection and AIDS. *MMWR.* 1987;36:509–515.

7. Minkoff HL, DeHovitz JA. Care of women infected with the human immunodeficiency virus. *JAMA.* 1991;266:2253–2258.

8. Musher DM, Hamill RJ, Baughn RE. Effect of human immunodeficiency virus (HIV) infection on the course of syphilis and on the response to treatment. *Ann Intern Med.* 1990;113:872–881.

9. Nanda D. Human immunodeficiency virus infection in pregnancy. *Obstet Gynecol Clin North Am.* 1990;17: 617–626.

10. Shayne VT, Kaplan BJ. Double victims: Poor women and AIDS. *Women & Health.* 1991;17:21–37.

Chapter Fourteen

....

....

....

....

Evaluation of Adult Patients Infected with HIV

RICHARD D. MUMA, PA-C
MICHAEL J. BORUCKI, MD
BARBARA ANN LYONS, MA, PA-C
RICHARD B. POLLARD, MD

Infection with HIV progresses to AIDS in at least 35% percent of those infected. Estimates place the number of people infected in the United States at a minimum of 1,000,000 people, and, at present, well over 200,000 cases of AIDS have been reported in the United States. In areas of high endemicity, the resources of available specialists have already been overwhelmed by the rapidly growing pool of patients. Consequently, primary health care workers, rather than specialists, are increasingly involved in

Reprinted with permission from *Phys Assist* 1991;15(1):23–32 and *Phys Assist* 1991;15(2):15,19–22.

the care of HIV-infected individuals. As the epidemic continues, primary care health care workers will need an increased understanding of the evaluation and management of patients with HIV.

The opportunistic infections and cancers that AIDS patients develop are not commonly seen in other patient populations. Also, multiple medical complications often occur simultaneously, resulting in a bewildering array of new and unusual medical problems. In addition to these medical complications, severe social, economic, and psychological problems complicate the care of these individuals.

The medical literature has focused on these issues as well as the epidemiology, immunology, and primary and secondary therapeutics in patients with AIDS, but very little attention has been directed to the initial and subsequent evaluations of asymptomatic or minimally symptomatic adult patients. This chapter will attempt to address some of these issues.

Once an individual has been diagnosed with HIV, the initial evaluation should be undertaken as rapidly as possible. The initial and subsequent evaluations require the following approach.

- Evaluation of the immune system and classification by CDC grouping (Table 14–1).
- Identification and treatment of infectious and neoplastic complications.
- Initiation of approved antiretroviral therapy.
- Consideration of experimental measures.

This particular methodology will allow the clinician to rapidly evaluate the immune system and identify treatable HIV-related disease processes so that either conventional chemotherapy or experimental chemotherapy can be instituted as soon as possible.

Recent evidence suggests that early evaluation of individuals infected with HIV is of increased benefit

TABLE 14–1. 1993 REVISED CLASSIFICATION SYSTEM FOR HIV INFECTION AND EXPANDED AIDS SURVEILLANCE DEFINITION FOR ADOLESCENTS AND ADULTS[a]

	Clinical Categories		
CD4 T-cell Categories	(A) Asymptomatic, acute (primary) HIV or PGL[b]	(B) Symptomatic, not (A) or (C) conditions[c]	(C) AIDS-indicator conditions[d]
(1) Greater than or equal to 500/mm³	A1	B1	C1
(2) 200–499/mm³	A2	B2	C2
(3) Less than 200/mm³; AIDS indicator T-cell count	A3	B3	C3

[a]C1–3, A3, and B3 illustrate the expanded AIDS surveillance case definition. Persons with AIDS-indicator conditions (categories C1-C3) as well as those with CD4 T-lymphocyte counts less than 200/mm³ (categories A3 and B3) are now reportable as AIDS cases in the Unites States and territories, effective January 1, 1993.

[b]PGL, persistent generalized lymphadenopathy. Clinical category A includes acute (primary) HIV infection.

[c]Examples include bacillary angiomatosis, oral candidiasis, vulvovaginal candidiasis, cervical dysplasia, cervical carcinoma in situ, constitutional symptoms or diarrhea lasting longer than 1 month, oral hairy leukoplakia, herpes zoster involving at least two distinct episodes or more than one dermatome, idiopathic thrombocytopenia, listeriosis, pelvic inflammatory disease, peripheral neuropathy.

[d]A list of these conditions can be found in Chapter 2.

Note: For classification purposes, category B conditions take precedence over those in category A, and category C conditions take precedence over category B. For example, someone treated for persistent vaginal candidiasis but who has now developed *P. carinii* pneumonia will remain in category C.

Adapted from the Centers for Disease Control and Prevention. 1993 revised classification system for HIV infection and expanded surveillance case definition for AIDS among adolescents and adults. *MMWR.* 1992;41(RR-17):1–19.

TABLE 14–2. HIV RISK GROUPS

Sexually active individuals who practice unprotected sex

Injecting drug users who share needles

Hemophiliacs and blood transfusion recipients who received
blood products prior to April 1985

Sexual partners and children of the above

---

through earlier identification and treatment with anti-retroviral drugs. For example, zidovudine (ZDV or AZT) has been demonstrated in National Institute of Health trials to have a statistically significant benefit when compared to placebo in patients with early HIV infection.[1,2] These results are encouraging and should prompt individuals at risk (Table 14–2) to obtain early HIV testing, evaluation, and intervention.

■ Evaluation of the Patient

When a patient is suspected to be HIV positive or has been diagnosed with the HIV infection, a baseline evaluation should be performed to determine the extent of the primary disease and diagnose secondary complications. The initial visit should consist of a thorough history and physical exam, baseline laboratory evaluation, patient education, and a psychosocial evaluation.

History

The history is the most important aspect of the evaluation, as it will suggest specific diagnostic and therapeutic interventions beyond the "baseline" evaluation. Although the history may be lengthy, it is important to identify and record those aspects of the medical history that may be individual baseline parameters to help differentiate them from those related to HIV.[3] The most important aspects of the history includes HIV risk factors, past medical history (especially sexually transmitted and injecting drug use diseases), and a thorough review of systems.

Risk Factors

Information obtained from the patient should first include risk factors for acquiring HIV such as homosexual activity, injecting drug use, and parenteral inoculation of body fluids (Table 14–2). Obtaining the risk factor from the patient is not only for epidemiological purposes, but also helps to identify special complications inherent to a particular risk group. For instance, homosexual patients often find themselves isolated from their family, friends, and significant others when the diagnosis becomes known. If this information is obtained early in the history, these stresses may be more readily recognized, and appropriate psychological referral can be made as needed. Patients at risk because of IDU may continue to abuse drugs and need referral to a drug treatment program. This information may help explain and potentially alleviate problems such as patient noncompliance with follow-up frequently seen with IDUs.

Medical History

A history of sexually transmitted diseases (STDs) including chancroid, condyloma, herpes, gonorrhea, and syphilis should also be obtained. Information regarding the treatment of syphilis is particularly important in this population, given the high occurrence of latent and neurosyphilis, and should include the agent, route, and duration of treatment.

A history of other disease processes such as tuberculosis, salmonellosis, zoster, and hepatitis B should be obtained from the patient, since these diseases may also impart significant morbidity.

Other disease processes may appear in association with immunosuppression; in particular, inquiries should be made regarding a history of any recurrent or unusual infections such as[3]:

- Tuberculosis, zoster, nocardiosis, genitorectal herpes
- Acute and chronic skin disorders such as molluscum contagiosum, folliculitis, venereal warts, seborrheic dermatitis, and fungal infections
- Oral, vaginal, or rectal candidiasis
- Diarrhea caused by *Giardia lamblia, Entamoeba histolytica, Salmonella, Shigella,* or *Campylobacter*
- Bacterial pneumonia, aseptic meningitis, sinusitis

A history of any of these infections may suggest a subtle impairment in immunity and, if such problems have occurred remotely, this may suggest long-standing immune impairment potentially attributable to HIV infection.

■ Review of Systems

Next, the history should focus on a review of body systems to screen for previously undiagnosed or intercurrent illnesses. Before particular systems are assessed, a general review of systems should be done. Inquiry should be made regarding weight loss, weakness, fatigue, fever, chills, and night sweats. These general symptoms may not be specific for a particular disease, but more often than not, one or all of them will be present if an infectious process or neoplasm is developing. The body systems targeted should routinely include those systems that are most often involved by the infectious or neoplastic complications that occur in HIV-infected individuals. These include the central nervous system, respiratory, cardiovascular, genitourinary and gastrointestinal systems, and the skin.

Direct inquiry should be made of 17 "cardinal" symptoms at the initial and at each follow-up visit. This list, although not intended to be exhaustive, may rather serve as an example of an abbreviated review of systems that allows for rapid screening for the major complications of HIV infection in symptomatic individuals. These symptoms are the very minimum that should be asked about at every visit.

The 17 symptoms and some of their associated differential considerations are presented in Box 14–1.

Because of the diverse pathology referable to the central nervous system (CNS), gastrointestinal system (GI), and pulmonary system, these three organ systems warrant special attention.

Central nervous system symptoms are frequently problematic in that baseline symptoms such as chronic headaches and symptoms specifically referable to HIV are often difficult to separate. A chronic headache could be little more than chronic tension headaches but could be one manifestation of an intracranial neoplasm or abscess. A careful review of systems may offer focal or localizing symptomatology to support a mass lesion, for example, diplopia, blurred vision, seizures, unilateral weakness, dysarthria, or a change in personality. CNS symptoms may be broadly divided into those that typically present with meningeal findings, those with focal findings, and those that are infrequently associated with focality of symptoms or exam. Intracranial focal processes include toxoplasmosis, non-Hodgkin's lymphoma, herpes encephalitis, and progressive multifocal leukoencephalopathy. Meningeal symptoms predominate with cryptococcal, tuberculous, or aseptic meningitis. The nonfocal dementing illnesses include primary HIV disease, syphilis, drug effects, electrolyte disturbances, hypoglycemia, and hypoxia.

Gastrointestinal symptoms may be broadly divided into an acute dysenteric pattern, with prominent fevers, abdominal pain, and a mucous to bloody diarrhea, and a

■ Box 14–1
Abbreviated Review of System

1. *Weight loss:* Opportunistic infection, tuberculosis, neoplasms, worsened malabsorptive diarrhea, depression, or as a CDC category C manifestation.

2. *Anorexia:* Hepatitis, carcinoma, disseminated opportunistic infection, AIDS dementia complex (ADC), metabolic disturbances such as diabetes, uremia, electrolyte abnormalities, depression, overuse of psychoactive pharmaceuticals, or illicit stimulant use.

3. *Increasing debility:* Neuromuscular complications of AIDS, AZT myopathy, steroid myopathy, ADC, Addison's disease, undiagnosed or spreading carcinoma, progressive multifocal leukoencephalopathy, cardiomyopathy, or overmedication.

4. *Adverse drug experiences:* Experimental therapeutics, "black market" remedies, over-the-counter drugs, or illicit drug use/abuse.

5. *Fevers:* Opportunistic infection (particularly *P. carinii*, disseminated fungi, mycobacterioses), infections with more "conventional" pathogens, non-Hodgkin's lymphoma, drug fever, or as a CDC category B manifestation of disease.

6. *Rigors:* Bacterial infections, catheter infections, phlebitis, endocarditis, mycobacteriosis, disseminated fungal opportunists, or malaria (if traveled or resided in an endemic area).

7. *Night sweats:* Tuberculosis, disseminated fungal infections, pyogenic infections, or lymphoma.

8. *Headache:* Meningitis (tuberculous, fungal, or aseptic), mass lesions (toxoplasmosis, nocardio-

— *continued* —

■ **Box 14–1** *(continued)*

sis, or lymphoma), or more "conventional" causes (tension, vascular, or cluster headaches).

9. *Change in vision:* Retinitis caused by cytomegalovirus or toxoplasmosis, ethambutol-induced optic neuritis, zoster ophthalmicus, or syphilitic, herpetic, fungal, or tuberculous involvement of the uveal tract.

10. *Diplopia:* Intracranial mass lesions from toxoplasmosis, nocardiosis, or lymphoma or extracranial involvement of the extraocular muscles.

11. *Dysphagia:* Esophageal involvement by *Candida*, herpes simplex virus, lymphoma, Kaposi's sarcoma, or AZT-induced erosions.

12. *Dyspnea:* Pulmonary involvement by *P. carinii*, cytomegalovirus, typical tuberculosis, atypical mycobacterioses, histoplasmosis, cryptococcoses, coccidioidomycosis, lymphoma, Kaposi's sarcoma, nonspecific interstitial pneumonitis, or edema from left ventricle failure.

13. *Diarrhea:* Salmonellosis, shigellosis, traveler's diarrhea, typical and atypical mycobacterioses, strongyloidiasis, giardiasis, amoebiasis, cryptosporidiosis, isosporiasis, cytomegalovirus, pseudomembranous colitis (following antimicrobial therapy), Addison's disease, malabsorption, excesses of caloric supplementation, hypervitaminosis D, or as a CDC category B manifestation.

14. *Changing lymphadenopathy:* CDC category A manifestation of disease if persistent and involving multiple noninguinal sites, lymphoma, "reactive" (in association with severe dermatitis),

— *continued* —

> pseudolymphoma (associated with phenytoin), cytomegalovirus or Epstein-Barr mononucleosis, toxoplasmosis, syphilis, or disseminated tuberculous or fungal disease.
>
> 15. *Oral lesions:* Thrush, oral hairy leukoplakia, histoplasmosis, herpes simplex, aphthous lesions, Kaposi's sarcoma.
> 16. *Rashes:* Seborrheic dermatitis, papular eruption of HIV, tinea, scabies, secondary syphilis, zoster, disseminated herpes simplex, folliculitis, disseminated fungal infections, Kaposi's sarcoma, thrombocytopenia purpura, drug reaction (especially to sulfa antimicrobial, ampicillin, amoxicillin, and phenytoin).
> 17. *Change in mental status:* AIDS dementia complex, intracranial mass lesions, progressive multifocal leukoencephalopathy, neurosyphilis, *Toxoplasma* encephalitis, herpes encephalitis, meningitis, Addison's disease, metabolic aberrations (electrolyte, glucose, uremia, hypoxia, acidosis), Wernicke's encephalopathy, sepsis, psychoactive drug excess.

chronic pattern, with diarrhea present for in excess of 2 weeks without associated fevers and without an abrupt change in volume or frequency. Dysenteric illness suggests the classical diarrheal pathogens of the immunocompetent host: salmonellosis, shigellosis, amoebiasis, traveler's diarrhea, and pseudomembranous colitis. Chronic diarrhea is more commonly a primary manifestation of HIV infection or caused by cryptosporidiosis, isosporiasis, atypical mycobacterioses, or malabsorption.

Pulmonary symptoms such as cough and dyspnea suggest a wide range of processes that may be broadly divided into those that are frequently associated with fevers and those that are not. All the opportunistic infections, whether fungal, viral, parasitic, or mycobacterial in origin, are typically associated with fevers. By contrast, intrapulmonary disease from Kaposi's sarcoma or non-Hodgkin's lymphoma, or compromised left ventricular function from cardiomyopathy are uncommonly associated with fevers.

■ Physical Examination

The physical exam should be thorough and directed toward the body systems discussed previously. Thus, the major foci of the physical examination of the HIV-positive patient should include the mouth, eyes, skin, central and peripheral nervous system, lungs, heart, lymph nodes, abdomen, rectum, and genitalia.

Mouth

When inspecting the mouth, particular attention should be given to white plaques on the buccal mucosa, soft and hard palates, and the tongue. White, plaque-like lesions are most commonly oral *Candida* but may represent oral hairy leukoplakia. Oral hairy leukoplakia usually develops on the lateral aspects of the tongue, and, unlike oral *Candida,* oral hairy leukoplakia is not easily removed by scraping. Other common oral findings in the mouth include ulcerative lesions, which may indicate herpes simplex, aphthous ulcers, or histoplasmosis. Purple, brown, raised lesions in the oral cavity should be considered Kaposi's sarcoma until proven otherwise (see Chapter 12).

Eyes

Clinical abnormalities that can occur can be caused by microvascular abnormalities such as cotton wool spots.

Cytomegalovirus and Kaposi's sarcoma are also common. Less common causes include toxoplasmosis, herpes simplex, zoster, *Cryptococcus, Candida, Mycobacterium avium-intracellulare,* and tuberculosis.

Of these possibilities, cytomegalovirus retinitis remains the most common cause of vision loss in AIDS patients. Funduscopic findings usually consist of extensive perivascular exudates and hemorrhages. Cotton wool spots may also be associated with active retinitis. According to one source, cytomegalovirus retinitis typically affects the more immune-debilitated patients.[4] This observation is supported by the finding that the infection rate is as high as 35% in several autopsy series but as low as 5% in the ambulatory population. An important feature of cytomegalovirus retinitis, which distinguishes it from toxoplasmosis, candidiasis, and other causes, is the frequent absence of vitreous inflammatory response. In cytomegalovirus retinitis, the retina is easily visualized.

Extraretinal ocular disease is most commonly caused by Kaposi's sarcoma. Kaposi's sarcoma most commonly involves the skin, but mucosal disease may involve the gastrointestinal tract, oropharynx, or conjunctival structures.[5] Although Kaposi's sarcoma, in this particular presentation, does not usually cause significant discomfort or pain, it does commonly cause unacceptable cosmeses.

Skin

Examination of the skin is challenging because common skin disorders may present in an exaggerated manner, making them difficult to diagnose. Common skin lesions include herpes simplex, herpes zoster, condyloma, abscess formation (particularly perirectal abscesses), folliculitis, secondary syphilis, scabies, paronychia/onycholysis, tinea versicolor, Kaposi's sarcoma, seborrheic dermatitis, and xerosis.[6] These present more often in individuals with a compromised immune system (T4 cell count less than 200/mm^3). In addition, patients with T4 count less than 200/mm^3 may have lesions that present atypically such as severe ulcerative lesions caused by herpes simplex.

Central and Peripheral Nervous System

Neurologic manifestations, both central and peripheral, occur commonly; therefore, close attention should be focused toward the neurologic exam. A complete neurologic exam should be done, including evaluation of the cranial nerves, motor and sensory systems, reflexes, gait, station, cerebral function, and special maneuvers such as testing for meningeal signs (Brudzinski's and Kernig's), and frontal release signs (grasp reflex and snout reflex). When indicated, referral for a neuropsychological exam should be considered, especially when a cognitive/motor/behavioral disorder is suspected, as in ADC. To complicate matters, distinct as well as subtle changes may be seen on these exams.

The most common neurologic manifestation in AIDS patients is ADC.[7–10] The changes seen are mild at the beginning and progress throughout the course of the disease to a more severe state. These changes may be difficult to distinguish from other causes of neurologic dysfunction. Early in the course of the disease, there may be impairment in both verbal and motor response seen on the exam. At this point, slurred speech and difficulty coordinating hand movements may be observed. The impairment is more obvious when the disease has progressed over several months. With progression, motor exam abnormalities may show slowing of finger opposition, wrist rotation, and foot tapping. Much later in the course of the disease, ataxia and clumsiness may progress to paraparesis and urinary/fecal incontinence. Neuropsychological exam abnormalities become apparent as ADC progresses and include difficulty in short-term memory and attention as manifest by difficulty with performing serial 7s, 2 and 7 test, digit span, and symbol-digit tests.

Secondary neurologic manifestations may be easier to diagnose because they more commonly cause symptomatology. Diseases such as central nervous system toxoplasmosis, primary brain lymphoma, herpes encephalitis, and progressive multifocal leukoencephalopathy typically present with focal deficits.[7] Cryptococcal meningitis, aseptic meningitis, and neurosyphilis may have focal findings as well, but will often have a subacute presentation with more mild findings such as meningeal signs and altered mental status.

Vacuolar myelopathy may also occur and should be differentiated from other causes of CNS dysfunction. This degenerative condition, in which an open space forms in the spinal cord tissue, is characterized by a progressive spastic paraparesis and upper motor neuron deficits. Ataxia and hyperreflexia have also been described.

Peripheral manifestations caused by HIV include sensory neuropathies and inflammatory demyelinating polyneuropathies. Patients often describe paresthesias, painful dysesthesias, and muscle weakness in the extremities. However, in the latter case, the weakness may be generalized. Neurologic exam findings may show mild to marked motor deficits and absent or decreased reflexes.

Lungs

As a group, pulmonary diseases cause the majority of morbidity and mortality in patients with AIDS. Index diagnosis and recurrences of *P. carinii,* in particular, are common. Other opportunistic organisms that cause pulmonary infections include cytomegalovirus, typical tuberculosis, atypical mycobacterioses, histoplasmosis, cryptococcosis, and coccidioidomycosis.[11] Neoplasms and lymphoproliferative disorders such as lymphoma, Kaposi's sarcoma, and lymphoid interstitial pneumonitis can also cause pulmonary disease. Careful examination of the lungs including auscultation of the lungs for wheezing and crackles should be routinely performed, especially when there is a history from the patient of nonproductive cough, fever, dyspnea, or tachypnea.

Heart

Cardiovascular complications of HIV are uncommon. Tuberculosis and other fungal organisms may cause pericardial effusions; thus, a complex cardiac exam should be done. A more worrisome problem, particularly in intravenous drug users, is the possibility of bacterial endocarditis. A cardiomyopathy has been associated with HIV, and although uncommon, it connotes a very poor prognosis.

Lymph Nodes

Inspection of lymph nodes should be considered routine since many of the AIDS-defining illnesses can cause enlarged lymph nodes. Changes in lymph nodes can be associated with viruses, specifically CMV, EBV, and HIV. As a general rule, soft, mobile, and tender nodes have viral etiologies, whereas firm, tender, or fixed nodes may indicate problematic secondary processes such as bacterial, fungal, or mycobacterial infections or neoplasm. Hard, fixed, and nontender nodes usually indicate neoplastic involvement. One should be concerned especially if the nodes begin to change (increase in size or become asymmetrical). Nodes that should be surveyed include supraclavicular, posterior, and anterior cervical, pre- and postauricular, tonsillar, occipital, submandibular, submental, epitrochlear, axillary, femoral, and inguinal.

Abdomen

The abdomen should be inspected for masses, organomegaly, ascites, and tenderness. Hepatosplenomegaly may be associated with viral hepatitis, disseminated fungal, or mycobacterial infections. Masses or extensive organomegaly usually indicate neoplastic or fungal involvement. Most commonly, in patients with diarrhea, a nondescript pain is elicited on the exam, usually in the lower quadrants, and may indicate a colitis caused by parasites, bacteria, or viruses. Malabsorption may also cause diarrhea without associated physical findings. Ascites may complicate prominent hepatic involvement by fungi, tuberculous and nontuberculous mycobacterioses, Kaposi's sarcoma, or lymphoma.

Genitalia and Rectum

Both the genitalia and rectum should be inspected and palpated for lesions consistent with herpes, scabies, syphilis, tinea, chancroid, condyloma, and Kaposi's sarcoma. All but the latter are frequently seen in these areas. Kaposi's sarcoma may be seen in the later stages of the disease. A rectal exam should be performed in all patients. In men, prostatitis and proctitis should be looked for; in both sexes, a stool test for occult blood to rule out gastrointestinal bleeding should be performed.

■ Laboratory and Diagnostic Evaluation

In concert with the goals of performing a complete history and physical examination, the laboratory studies stress the rapid evaluation and the early identification of concurrent illnesses. It is believed that early intervention and treatment may improve the long-term survival of patients infected with HIV. Thus, patients may be evaluated as one of two major groups as defined by history and physical exam (Table 14–3).

TABLE 14–3. LABORATORY AND DIAGNOSTIC EVALUATION AT THE UNIVERSITY OF TEXAS MEDICAL BRANCH, GALVESTON, TEXAS

Asymptomatic Patients at Risk for HIV
CBC with differential
Liver transaminases (SGOT/SGPT)
Syphilis screen (RPR or VDRL), confirmation by FTA-ABS
HIV ELISA and Western blot confirmation
Prior exposure hepatitis panel

Symptomatic and HIV Positive and/or Suspected to Have an AIDS-Related Condition
CBC with differential
Liver transaminases (SGOT/SGPT)
Syphilis screen (RPR or VDRL), confirmation by FTA-ABS
Serology for CMV, EBV, HSV, toxoplasmosis, cryptococcus
Prior exposure hepatitis panel
T4/T8 subsets
Beta-2 microglobulin
Fungal immunodiffusion titer
Chest x-ray
Electroencephalogram

The two major groups are:

- Asymptomatic patients and at-risk patients for HIV
- Symptomatic and HIV positive and/or suspected to have an AIDS-related condition

The first group will most likely include an abbreviated laboratory evaluation, whereas symptomatic individuals or those with known AIDS will require a more extensive work-up.

Asymptomatic and High Risk

If patients are at risk for the HIV infection but their antibody status is unknown, they should be screened for HIV using the enzyme immunoassay (EIA) to detect HIV antibodies.[12,13] Confirmation of HIV antibodies can be followed up with a Western blot. (Note: seronegative patients must be counseled that testing does not substitute for prevention of AIDS; continued high-risk behavior poses a hazard regardless of the frequency of testing). At-risk patients as well as known seropositives should be screened for sexually transmitted diseases, hepatitis, and tuberculosis. A complete blood count (CBC) with differential should be routinely performed because of the increased incidence of anemia, thrombocytopenia, and neutropenia that occurs in the latter stages of HIV infection.[14] Serum for liver transaminases (SGOT and SGPT) and hepatitis (A, B, and C) is needed to assess ongoing liver function and prior/present infection with hepatitis, particularly hepatitis B.[15–17]

Evaluation for sexually transmitted diseases should begin with screening for syphilis with nontreponemal tests such as the RPR (rapid plasma reagin) or VDRL (venereal disease research laboratory) with a confirmatory FTA ABS (fluorescent treponemal antibody absorption) test as indicated. This is extremely important since there is an accelerated rate of neurosyphilis in HIV patients and apparent refractoriness to therapy.[18] Any suspicious lesion or discharge should be further evaluated for syphilis with dark-field microscopy and for *N. gonorrhea, Chlamydia,* and herpes simplex by appropriate culture. All patients should undergo PPD skin testing for tuberculosis as *M. tuberculosis* causes frequent morbidity in this patient population.

Symptomatic HIV Infection or AIDS

Any patients who have a social history and symptoms compatible with a disease associated with HIV should be evaluated using a separate protocol (Table 14–3) to screen for HIV-related illnesses and diagnose already existing conditions. Like the asymptomatic and high-risk individual, this group of patients should also have blood drawn for complete hemogram, liver transaminases, and hepatitis and syphilis serology. In addition, this group of patients should have virologic studies drawn that include serology for cytomegalovirus (CMV) and herpes simplex virus (HSV). Infections with HSV and CMV are common in patients at risk for AIDS.[19] Disease occurs following reactivation and may cause significant morbidity and mortality,[20] may adversely affect cell-mediated immunity,[21,22] and may augment infection with HIV.[23]

Determination of the absolute T4 cell number is the principal means of determining if sufficient immune dysfunction has occurred to warrant therapy, since most antiretroviral therapies like zidovudine (ZDV) are not initiated until some evidence for immunosuppression has occurred.[1,2,24] To evaluate the immune system, T4/T8 subsets and serum beta-2-microglobulin (B2M) should be obtained.

The absolute T4 cell number reflects the activity of HIV infection and, in concert with the B2M, is useful for prognosticating the patient's risk to progression to symptomatic disease.[25,26] In addition, the T4 cell plays a central role in the cell-mediated immune system. Defects in cell-mediated immunity allow for the development of diseases in patients with AIDS (*P. carinii, Toxoplasma gondii*, cytomegalovirus, and others). The T4/T8 ratio may be helpful as well and is usually inverted with advanced disease. The normal range for the absolute T4 count ranges between 500 and 1000/mm^3 but may vary somewhat from lab to lab. Most individuals do not develop opportunistic infections until the absolute T4 count drops consistently below 200/mm^3 and the B2M reaches levels above 3 mg/L.

Fungal studies are usually reserved for individuals who present with symptoms suggestive of a disseminated mycosis such as fevers of unknown etiology but can be obtained at baseline for future comparison. A fungal immunodiffusion is an inexpensive means of determining prior infection with common fungal organisms, such as histoplasmosis, cryptococcus, coccidioidomycosis, and blastomycosis. If a patient complains of a headache and fevers, a serum cryptococcal antigen may be a useful screening test.[27] The antigen appears to be a rapid, sensitive, and specific test for active disseminated cryptococcal disease. If a patient appears to have a fungal or acid-fast systemic fungal infection, bone marrow biopsies may be helpful by identifying organisms on stains or as isolates. Additional blood and urine cultures should be ordered for fungal isolates and acid-fast organisms.

Another baseline study should include a toxoplasmosis titer, since disease caused by toxoplasmosis also occurs principally through reactivation of an old infection. This organism most commonly causes abscess formation or encephalitis[28] in the compromised host but can also cause retinitis[29] and pneumonitis.

Unfortunately, an elevated toxoplasmosis titer by itself is not diagnostic for an active infection, but is in a clinically compatible setting. For encephalitis, computerized tomography (CT) of the head to demonstrate ring enhancing lesions or a biopsy demonstrating infected brain tissue is needed. The latter is usually not indicated if the lesions decrease in size after appropriate treatment.

As mentioned earlier, symptoms suggestive of pulmonary disease should have special consideration.[30] Most of the diseases that patients encounter are pulmonary in nature. Whether the patient has pulmonary symptoms or not, a baseline chest x-ray should be ordered for comparison in the future and may be particularly useful if changes of old histoplasmosis or tuberculosis are present. This becomes important when minimal changes are seen on chest films even in the presence of an active pulmonary infection. Special attention should be taken when a diffuse interstitial pattern is seen on a chest x-ray. Organisms such as *P. carinii,* CMV, and histoplasmosis should be included in the differential. Other findings that should increase suspicion of an active pulmonary process include the presence of granulomata, cavities, and hilar enlargement. Any of these findings may suggest a mycobacterial infection or fungal infections such as histoplasmosis, although pneumatocele associated with PCP may mimic cavitary disease. The definitive diagnosis of any uncertain chest x-ray abnormality should be made by bronchoscopy with a bronchoalveolar lavage (BAL).[31,32]

Occasionally, transbronchial biopsy is necessary to define more focal disease. Sputum analysis may be helpful if pulmonary tuberculosis is suspected but is less useful when diseases such as *P. carinii,* CMV, and fungal infections, such as histoplasmosis, are present. An arterial blood gas may be helpful to determine the extent of hypoxia and may prompt empiric treatment while awaiting definitive diagnosis. Generally, if the PO_2 is less than 60 mm Hg, empiric therapy for PCP should be started and continued until the patient stabilizes. The diagnosis can be confirmed using bronchoscopy with BAL since the organisms will still be readily identifiable on smear following a short course of therapy. An example may include a patient with fever, severe dyspnea, dry cough, a chest x-ray showing diffuse interstitial infiltrates, and a PO_2 of 55 mm Hg. The diagnosis is most likely PCP with severe hypoxia. In this clinical situation, therapy should not be delayed while awaiting bronchoscopy; therefore, empiric therapy with trimethropim-sulfamethoxazole or pentamidine should be initiated.[33] If there is not a significant amount of hypoxia and the patient is clinically stable, a bronchoscopy should be obtained first for the diagnosis.

Like pulmonary infections, diarrhea also causes significant morbidity in patients with HIV and deserves equal attention.[34,35] If a patient presents with a history of diarrhea that does not resolve spontaneously, evaluation of the cause is indicated. Pathogens causing diarrhea in HIV patients are broad and may include parasites, bacteria, or viruses. To define the etiology, samples should be obtained for ova and parasites, AFB smear, cryptosporidiosis, and culture for enteric pathogens such as *Salmonella, Shigella, Campylobacter,* mycobacteriosis, and *E. coli.* If the diarrhea persists and no pathogen is identified, then a barium enema can be obtained to look for mucosal abnormalities followed by endoscopy for biopsy of involved areas. Fortunately, most cases of diarrhea have confirmed etiologies by microbiologic evaluation of stool samples.

Another adjunct when initially evaluating the HIV-positive patient is the electroencephalogram (EEG). Since dementia associated with HIV is common, particularly in patients with full-blown AIDS, the EEG may be able to pick up early changes consistent with AIDS dementia complex. If dementia is present, the EEG may reveal mild to severe slowing of brain wave activity. Although not wholly diagnostic for ADC, an EEG may be more helpful in following the progression of the dementia. A more helpful diagnostic tool in diagnosis of ADC is a head CT: cerebral atrophy can be demonstrated in most cases of advanced ADC.

◼ Psychosocial Evaluation and Patient Education

Patients who have been diagnosed in any group or stage of the HIV infection may eventually begin to develop

TABLE 14–4. MODES OF HIV TRANSMISSION

Adult HIV Infection

Vaginal and/or receptive anal intercourse
Infection/percutaneous exposure with HIV-infected blood or
   blood products
Maternal–fetal transmission.

physical as well as psychosocial problems. Both of these issues are usually related and tend to rise and fall in level of importance in relation to the fear of the unknown. Some of the specific issues that patients will have to deal with include deteriorating health, treatment options, death and dying, loss of job and financial security, loss of emotional or family support, relationship problems, and changes in lifestyle (see Chapters 16 and 21).[36] It is important that the health care professional working with this population be extremely sensitive to these issues and be able to understand and identify the resources available to the client. Also at this point, there should be a discussion with the patient on HIV prevention. This can be accomplished by spending a brief amount of time at the end of each patient encounter. Minimum information to the patient should include discussion on modes of transmission (Table 14–4), protective measures, and safe sex (see Chapter 20).

References

1. Volberding PA, Lagakos SW, Koch MA, et al. Zidovudine in asymptomatic human immunodeficiency virus infection: a controlled trial in persons with fewer than 500 CD4-positive cells per cubic millimeter. *N Engl J Med.* 1990;322:941–949.

2. Fischl MA, Richman DD, Hansen N, et al. The safety and efficacy of zidovudine (AZT) in the treatment of subjects with mildly symptomatic human immunodeficiency virus type 1 (HIV) infection: a double-blind,

placebo-controlled trial. *Ann Intern Med.* 1990;112:727–737.

3. Clement M, Franke E, Wisniewski TL. Managing the HIV-positive patient. *Patient Care.* 1989;23:51–87.

4. Chess J, Fisher J. Ophthalmologic manifestations of AIDS. *Phys Assist.* 1989;13:130–135.

5. Odajynk C, Muggia FM. Treatment of Kaposi's sarcoma: overview and analysis by clinical setting. *J Clin Oncol.* 1985;3:1277–1285.

6. Kaplan MH, Sadick N, McNutt S, et al. Dermatologic findings and manifestations of acquired immunodeficiency syndrome. *J Am Acad Phys Assist.* 1988;1:91–108.

7. McArthur JH, Palenicek JG, Bowersox LL. Human immunodeficiency virus and the nervous system. *Nurs Clin North Am.* 1988;23:823–841.

8. Berger JR. Neurologic complications of human immunodeficiency virus infection. *Postgrad Med.* 1987;81:72–79.

9. Price RW, Sidtis J, Rosenblum M. The AIDS dementia complex: some current questions. *Ann Neurol.* 1988;23(suppl):27–33.

10. Navia BA, Jordan BD, Price RW. The AIDS dementia complex: I. clinical features. *Ann Neurol.* 1986;19:517–524.

11. Marchevsky A, Rosen MJ, Chrystal G, et al. Pulmonary complications of the acquired immunodeficiency syndrome: a clinicopathologic study of 70 cases. *Hum Pathol.* 1985;16:659–670.

12. Centers for Disease Control. Public Health Service guidelines for counseling and antibody testing to prevent HIV infection and AIDS. *MMWR.* 1987;36:509–515.

13. Centers for Disease Control. Interpretation and use of the Western blot assay for serodiagnosis of human immunodeficiency virus type-1 infections. *MMWR.* 1989;38:1–7.

14. Murphy MF, Metcalfe P, Waters AH, et al. Incidence and mechanism of neutropenia and thrombocytopenia in patients with human immunodeficiency virus infection. *Br J Haematol.* 1987;66:337–340.

15. Rustgi VK, Hoofnagle JH, Gerin JL, et al. Hepatitis B virus infection in the acquired immunodeficiency syndrome. *Ann Intern Med.* 1984;101:795–797.

16. Alter MJ, Hadler SC, Margolis HS, et al. The changing epidemiology of hepatitis B in the United States. *JAMA.* 1990;263:1218–1222.

17. McDonald JA, Caruso L, Karayiannis P, et al. Diminished responsiveness of male homosexual chronic hepatitis B virus carriers with HTLV-III antibodies to recombinant alpha-interferon. *Hepatology* 1987;7:719–723.

18. Centers for Disease Control. Sexually transmitted diseases treatment guidelines. *MMWR.* 1989;38:1–43.

19. Holmberg SD, Stewart JA, Gerber AR, et al. Prior herpes simplex virus type 2 infection as a risk factor for HIV infection. *JAMA.* 1988;259:1048–1050.

20. Suttman U, Willers H, Gerdelmann R, et al. Cytomegalovirus infection in HIV-1 infected individuals. *Infection.* 1988;16:111–114.

21. Schrier R, Rice G, Oldstone M. Suppression of natural killer cell activity and T cell proliferation by fresh isolates of human cytomegalovirus. *J Infect Dis.* 1986; 153:1084–1091.

22. Carney W, Rubin R, Hoffman R, et al. Analysis of T lymphocyte subsets in cytomegalovirus mononucleosis. *J Immunol.* 1981;126:2114–2116.

23. Mosca JD, Bednarik DP, Raj NBK, et al. Herpes simplex virus type-1 can reactivate transcription of latent human immunodeficiency virus. *Nature.* 1987;325:67–70.

24. AZT Collaborative Working Group. The efficacy of azidothymadine (AZT) in the treatment of patients

with AIDS-related complex. *N Engl J Med.* 1987;317:185–191.

25. de Wolf F, Roos M, Lange JMA, et al. Decline in CD4 cell numbers reflects increase in HIV-1 replication. *AIDS Res Hum Retroviruses.* 1988;4:433–440.

26. Moss AR, Bachetti P, Osmaond D, et al. Seropositivity for HIV and the development of AIDS or AIDS related condition: Three year followup of The San Francisco General Hospital Cohort. *Br Med J.* 1988;296:745–750.

27. Kovacs JA, Kovacs A, Polis M, et al. Cryptococcosis in the acquired immunodeficiency syndrome. *Ann Intern Med.* 1985;103:533–538.

28. Levy RM, Rosenbloom S, Perrett LV. Neuroradiologic findings in AIDS: a review of 200 cases. *Am J Roentgenol.* 1986; 147:977–983.

29. Friedman AH. The retinal lesions of the acquired immunodeficiency syndrome. *Trans Am Ophthal Soc.* 1984;82:447–492.

30. Murray JF, Garay SM, Hopewell PC, et al. Pulmonary complications of the acquired immunodeficiency syndrome: an update. Report of the second National Heart, Lung, and Blood Institute workshop. *Am Rev Respir Dis.* 1987;135:504–509.

31. Barrio JL, Harcup C, Baier HJ, et al. Value of repeat fiberoptic bronchoscopies and significance of nondiagnostic bronchoscopic results in patients with the acquired immunodeficiency syndrome. *Am Rev Respir Dis.* 1987;135:422–425.

32. Golden JA, Hollander H, Stulbarg MS, et al. Bronchoalveolar lavage as the exclusive diagnostic modality for *Pneumocystis carinii* pneumonia: a prospective study among patients with the acquired immunodeficiency syndrome. *Chest.* 1986;90:18–22.

33. Sattler FR, Cowan R, Nielsen DM, et al. Trimethoprim-sulfamethoxazole compared with pentamidine for

treatment of *Pneumocystis carinii* pneumonia in the acquired immunodeficiency syndrome: a prospective, noncrossover study. *Ann Intern Med.* 1988;109: 280–287.

34. Borich A, Kotler DP. Combating chronic diarrhea in AIDS patients. *Phys Assist.* 1990;14:101–114.

35. Soave R, Johnson WD. Cryptosporidium and *Isospora* infections. *J Infect Dis.* 1988;157:225–229.

36. Baker J, Muma RD. Counseling patients with HIV infection. *Phys Assist.* 1991;15(7):40–42, 47–48.

Chapter Fifteen

Pediatric HIV Infection

Karen S. Stephenson, PA-C

◼ The Epidemiology of Pediatric AIDS

The first pediatric case was identified in 1982. Through September, 1992, there have been 4051 cases reported with a steadily growing number of new cases per year.[1]

Children (those < 13 years of age) usually acquire the disease by perinatal routes, transfusion, and treatment of hemophilia. As of December, 1989, percentages for these means were 83%, 9%, and 5%, respectively. Another 3% of the infections have no determined cause.[2] Children may also acquire infection from sexual exposure, including assault.[3]

Three means of transmission between mother and child include placenta, contact with mother's blood at delivery, and breast feeding. Cesarean sections will not prevent infection at delivery.[2]

◼ Diagnosis

The mean age for diagnosis of perinatally infected children is 17 months. There are quite a variety of symptoms noted depending upon the age of the child at presentation

TABLE 15–1. CDC CLASSIFICATION FOR AIDS IN CHILDREN[4]

Class P-O. Indeterminate infection

Class P-1. Asymptomatic Infection

   Subclass A. Normal immune function

   Subclass B. Abnormal immune function

   Subclass C. Immune function not tested

Class P-2. Symptomatic infection

   Subclass A. Nonspecific findings

   Subclass B. Progressive neurologic disease

   Subclass C. Lymphoid interstitial pneumonitis

   Subclass D. Secondary infectious disease

      Category D-1 CDC definition of AIDS

      Category D-2 Recurrent serious bacterial infection

      Category D-3 Other infectious disease

   Subclass E. Secondary cancers

      Category E-1 CDC listing

      Category E-2 Other malignancies possibly associated with HIV

   Subclass F. Other diseases possibly due to HIV

(Table 15–1). Infants may demonstrate mucocutaneous candidiasis, failure to thrive, hepatosplenomegaly, or respiratory distress secondary to *P. carinii* pneumonia. Toddlers may have parotitis, generalized lymphadenopathy, recurrent bacterial infection, neurological disease, or development abnormalities. For older children, symptoms may include failure to thrive, hepatosplenomegaly, chronic interstitial pneumonia, or a combination of these.[3]

■ Laboratory Evaluation

T4 (helper) lymphopenia with decreased absolute numbers of T4 lymphocytes and an inverted T4:T8 ratio are hallmarks of HIV infection. However, children with HIV

TABLE 15–2. T4 LYMPHOCYTE PARAMETERS FOR NORMAL, HEALTHY CHILDREN AND ADULTS[5]

	1–6 mo.	7–12 mo.	13–24 mo.	25–74 mo.	Adults
Number tested	106	28	46	29	327
Absolute T4+ count					
Median cells/mm^3	3211	3128	2601	1668	1027
5–95 percentile (cells/mm^3)	1153–5285	967–5289	739–4463	505–2831	237–1817
Percentage T4+ cells					
Median (%)	51.6	47.9	45.8	42.1	50.9
5–95 percentile (%)	36.3–67.1	32.8–63.0	31.2–60.4	32.2–52.0	34.7–67.1
T4:T8 Ratio					
Median	2.2	2.1	2.0	1.4	1.7
5–95 percentile	0.9–3.5	0.8–3.4	0.6–3.4	0.7–2.1	0.4–3.0

infection may have a normal T4 cell count. B cells may also undergo change; commonly there is hypergammaglobulinemia, but the opposite may occur as well.[3] Table 15–2 contains age-specific normal T4 counts.

■ HIV Testing in Children

Detection of HIV infection in infants is difficult because the child passively acquires antibodies from the mother. These maternal antibodies may last for as long as 18 months,[6] but uninfected children usually revert to a negative status around 9 to 10 months.[3]

Because the maternal antibodies are of the IgG class, efforts at testing have been directed toward measuring the infant's evidence of infection. This is particularly important to the infant because decisions about treatment must be made as soon as possible, and there are risks with administration of zidovudine (AZT). The potential benefits for early treatment to the infant were recently identified by the American Academy of Pediatrics. These include reduced morbidity, dissemination of information regarding the risk of HIV transmission from breast milk and during subsequent pregnancies, and possible further transmission sexually by the mother and the father.[7]

The decision about early treatment is complicated by the fact that only a third of infants exposed to the virus perinatally become infected. The estimates range from 12.9% to 39%,[6] and the remaining infants gradually clear the mother's IgG antibodies from their bloodstreams.[3]

There are presently five means of evaluating an infant for signs of an infection. These include detecting HIV-specific antigen (HIV p24 antigen ELISA), demonstrating production of HIV-specific antibodies by the patient's lymphocytes in vitro, detecting HIV-specific DNA using the polymerase chain reaction, detecting anti-HIV IgA antibodies, or demonstrating the virus itself by culture.[8]

One method available for HIV testing is detection of p24 antigen. This antigen is a protein from the virion, but two problems exist with the test: p24 may not be present in asymptomatic patients,[3] and it may not be detectable in the presence of high levels of HIV-specific antibodies.[8]

Blood thought to contain the HIV virus can be cultured to detect the presence of lymphocytes producing antibodies, not the antibodies themselves. This is known as an in vitro production assay, or IVPA, and a product known as Elispot is available for IVPA testing. Maternal antibodies may interfere with this test, or there may be a false-negative result during asymptomatic periods when no antibodies are produced by activated lymphocytes.[8]

A new assay under development is measurement of HIV-DNA polymerase chain reactions (PCR). This DNA is incorporated into the human DNA by HIV. Because it is a relatively small amount of DNA, it must be amplified for measurement. Because DNA, rather than antibodies, is measured, this test provides a more specific test for the infection but is not very sensitive during the neonatal period. The results can be obtained in 1 day and only require a small amount of blood. Because of the small amounts of DNA measured, though, it is possible to have contamination from other studies (ie, measure DNA that actually belongs to another person) unless great care is taken in performing the test.[8]

The antibody assay used for adults detects IgG class antibodies, but that measurement is not appropriate for infants. Attention has now been directed toward antibodies produced by the infant, including IgM and IgA antibodies.[8] Evaluation of these two antibodies indicates that IgA measurements will be a more reliable test. IgG from the mother can block binding of IgA and IgM, but IgA persists in the baby's blood longer than IgM. This testing for IgA is presently not reliable for infants less than 3 months of age because evaluations have revealed that

IgA antibodies are frequently not present before 3 months of age.[9]

Viral cultures are also available. They take 7 to 28 days to complete and represent a significant risk to those monitoring the culture. They are also expensive and detect an infection in a newborn about 50% of the time.[8]

In summary, all of these methods are improving abilities to identify an HIV infection in children but are the least sensitive for newborns (those infants to 2 months of age). The PCR and viral cultures detect 50% of infections during this period whereas HIV-specific IgA and p24 assays are positive for fewer than 10% of newborns. In vitro antibody production is also not reliable during this period. On the other hand, most assays (PCR < IVAP < IgA, and culture) have 75% to 100% sensitivities by 6 months of age.[8]

■ Infectious Complications of HIV Infection in Children

Pulmonary complications include *Pneumocystis carinii* pneumonia (PCP), lymphoid interstitial pneumonia, tuberculosis (TB), and respiratory syncytial virus.[3] As in adults, PCP is the leading AIDS-indicator disease, and lymphoid interstitial pneumonia is the second most common in children. This second disease is not part of the syndrome associated with AIDS in adolescents and adults[10] (see Table 15–3).

Pneumocystis carinii Pneumonia

PCP presents with fever, a nonproductive cough, and tachypnea. Interstitial changes and air bronchograms can be seen on chest x-ray. The diagnosis is made by identifying characteristic cysts in respiratory secretions. Some children, though, will require bronchoscopy or lung bi-

TABLE 15–3. LEADING AIDS-INDICATOR DISEASES REPORTED IN CHILDREN FOR 1992[10]

Pneumocystis carinii pneumonia	31%
Lymphoid interstitial pneumonia and/or pulmonary lymphoid hyperplasia*	20%
HIV wasting syndrome	16%
HIV encephalopathy (dementia)	15%
Bacterial infections, multiple or recurrent*	13%
Candidiasis of esophagus	10%
Cytomegalovirus disease other than retinitis	7%
Mycobacterium avium or *M. kansasii*, disseminated or extrapulmonary	5%

These data are based on the 771 pediatric cases reported to the CDC for 1992. Adapted by permission of the *New England Journal of Medicine*.
*These conditions are not indicators for AIDS in adolescents or adults.

opsy to establish the diagnosis. Trimethoprim-sulfamethoxazole is the treatment of choice in children. Children have fewer side effects with this regimen than do adults, and pentamidine carries significant risks including hypoglycemia, pancreatitis, and renal failure.[3]

Treatment for children with PCP is TMP (20 mg/kg per day) and SMX (100 mg/kg per day) in four divided daily doses intravenously for 21 days. If TMP-SMX is not appropriate for a patient, intravenous pentamidine (4 mg/kg per day) in one daily dose for 12 to 14 days can be used. However, pentamidine has a high rate (50% to 60%) of adverse side effects. Pentamidine can be given intramuscularly, but painful sterile abscesses may develop.[11]

It is also important to provide adequate nutrition and pulmonary support for children with PCP. Children should be given 150 to 200 Cal/kg per day if they weigh less than 10 kg and 100 to 150 Cal/kg per day for children weighing more than 10 kg (1 Cal, or kilogram-calorie, equals 1000 cal). Children receive pulmonary support with intubation and mechanical ventilation based on their oxygen levels and the pH of the arterial blood.[11]

Lymphoid Interstitial Pneumonia

Lymphoid interstitial pneumonia (LIP) is a slowly progressive disorder with cough and mild hypoxemia. There is frequently a generalized adenopathy and salivary gland enlargement; digital clubbing is present in the late stages of the disease. A chest x-ray will show small nodules and fine reticular densities.[3] Sputum examination reveals lymphocytes, plasma cells, and macrophages.

Because there is no specific etiologic agent for LIP, treatment of the complications is as follows: administering the appropriate antimicrobial agent (bacterial or viral), oxygen, and bronchodilators as indicated. LIP has also improved after treatment with zidovudine.[12]

Tuberculosis

In the pediatric patient, tuberculosis is not yet associated frequently with the HIV infection as it is in adults, but TB is expected to become more common. This is, in part, because of the difficulties in confirming the diagnosis of tuberculosis in children. During the years 1985 to 1988, 90% of adults with TB were confirmed bacteriologically, whereas only 28% of children less then 15 years of age were.[13] In addition, several factors may cause the skin test to be falsely negative; these include a period of nonreactivity 10 weeks after HIV-infected persons contract TB, persons with recent live virus immunizations (MMR),[14] and being in the newborn age group.

Tuberculosis infections and HIV infections in children follow a pattern opposite that noted in adults. In adults, the tuberculin bacillus is usually acquired when the person is immunocompetent and represents an activation of a latent disease, whereas the child is usually infected with HIV in utero or perinatally. Because the child's immune system is not competent when TB is contracted, there may not be a positive skin test, pleural effusion, or lymphadenopathy.[13]

Children usually acquire their infection from members of their household, and the parent or parents at risk to transmit the HIV infection are also at risk for tuberculosis. Children with HIV and/or tuberculosis could be identified by careful follow-up of the contacts of an adult with tuberculosis. This surveillance is important because children may have nonspecific symptoms. Constitutional symptoms such as low-grade fever, cough, weight loss, night sweats, and failure to thrive may occur; other pulmonary symptoms are usually absent. Those pulmonary symptoms that have been observed with TB include wheezing, decreased breath sounds, tachypnea, and respiratory distress. These symptoms result from bronchial obstruction.[15]

The chest x-ray, on the other hand, may reveal substantial pathology. The initial infection may cause no visible changes, though hilar adenopathy may develop. In most children, the hilar adenopathy resolves, but in others, the adenopathy may lead to bronchial obstruction, perforation of the bronchus, and caseation. With proper treatment (isoniazid, rifampin, and pyrazinamide), these changes usually resolve.[15]

Respiratory Syncytial Virus

Respiratory syncytial virus (RSV) is a common respiratory infection in infants and young children, and most infections occur during fall and early spring. The usual clinical course includes 1 to 2 days of rhinitis, dry cough, mild to moderate fever, and the symptoms usually resolve in 3 to 7 days. Thirty to 40% of children go on to develop pneumonia and bronchiolitis; this then leads to signs of respiratory distress including cyanosis, tachypnea, inspiratory rales and expiratory wheezing, retractions, and cough.[16]

Radiographic findings include hyperinflation, increased bronchial markings, or pneumonia. The diagnosis can be confirmed by rapid antigen testing. Arterial blood gases are needed to assess the severity of respiratory distress, and hospitalization may be necessary. These children may need antiviral therapy with ribavirin by infant oxygen hood.[16] A small-particle aerosol generator (Viratek SPAG-2) should be used to provide the medication for 12 to 18 hours a day at a rate of 190 µg/L of air for at least 3 days and no longer than 7 days. The vial (6 g/vial) of ribavirin (Virazole) is diluted into sterile water and given with the aerosol generator that accompanies the medicine. Side effects from this drug include hypotension, cardiac arrest, digitalis toxicity, anemia, reticulocytosis, rash, conjunctivitis, and worsening of respiratory status. This drug is reserved for patients with severe lower-tract RSV infections.

Children who are HIV positive or who have AIDS also experience the spectrum of response to an RSV infection. Most children tolerate the infection without complications, but children with concurrent pneumonia or PCP infection are more likely to develop respiratory distress or failure and may require antiviral therapy.[3]

■ Congenital Syphilis and AIDS

In addition to acquiring an HIV infection from their mothers, infants may also be exposed to other sexually transmitted diseases. These include syphilis, gonorrhea, and hepatitis B infections.[3] In addition, the numbers of congenital syphilis cases reported to the CDC have been rising rapidly since 1986.[17] Two thirds or more of infants exposed to untreated syphilis become infected, and 38% to 64% of these infants are asymptomatic.[18]

There are a wide variety of findings associated with congenital syphilis. These variations are secondary to the maternal stage of syphilis, stage of pregnancy at the time of infection, rapidity of maternal diagnosis and treatment, adequacy of the maternal treatment for the fetus, maternal reinfection, and immunologic reaction of the fetus.[19]

The most common signs of congenital syphilis are condylomata lata, periostitis or osteochondritis, persistent rhinorrhea, and other manifestations listed in Table 15–4. Some of these signs are shared with infection with HIV. The classical signs of congenital syphilis do not appear until age 2 years or later.[19]

As for HIV infections in newborns, establishing the diagnosis is complicated by the maternal IgG antibodies to syphilis that cross the placenta. Despite this, prenatal screening remains the most important tool for treating the infection as quickly as possible, though pregnant women at greatest risk for syphilis may not seek prenatal care. Serum from the infant (rather than cord blood) should be analyzed for both VDRL and FTA ABS tests. Because of the maternal antibodies, the infant's VDRL should be at least fourfold that of the mother's titer. In addition, CSF analysis should be done with a nonquantitative VDRL test rather than rapid plasma reagin or FTA ABS. There is now an IgM antibody test that is particularly valuable for establishing the diagnosis when the mother's VDRL titer remains elevated or stable despite adequate treatment or when there is a discrepancy between the infant's and mother's titers. Confirmation of congenital syphilis can be done by dark-field testing of exudate or serum for *Treponema pallidum*.[19] Presumptive diagnosis can be established by criteria from the CDC[17] (Box 15–1).

Evaluation of congenital syphilis includes a thorough physical examination for any of the physical findings associated with this condition, long bone radiographs, simultaneous VDRL titers for mother and infant, con-

TABLE 15–4. CLINICAL FINDINGS OF CONGENITAL SYPHILIS[19]

Signs of Early Congenital Syphillis	Signs of Late Congenital Syphilis (After 2 yr)
Stillbirth	Frontal bossing
Funisitis	Short maxillae
Placentitis	Saddle nose
Enlarged placenta	Protruding mandible
Focal proliferative villitis	High-arched palate
Endovascular proliferation	Hutchinson teeth* (peg-shaped upper incisors)
Relative immaturity of villi	Mulberry molars
Nonimmune hydrops fetalis	Perioral fissures (rhagades)
Intrauterine growth retardation	Clutton joints (bilateral knee effusions)
Hepatosplenomegaly	Higoumenakis sign (sterno clavicular thickening)
With or without jaundice	Saber shins
Generalized lymphadenopathy	Flaring scapulas
Bone abnormalities	Interstitial keratitis*
Diaphyseal periostitis	Neurologic abnormalities
Osteochondritis	Mental retardation
Wimberger sign	Eighth cranial nerve deafness*
Mucocutaneous lesions	Hydrocephalus
Mucous patches	Mental retardation
Pigmented macules (condylomata lata)	
Vesiculobullous rash	
Any unexplained rash involving palms and soles	
Intractable diaper rash	
Persistent rhinitis (snuffles)	
Nephrotic syndrome	
Pneumonitis ("pneumonia alba")	
Neurologic abnormalities	
Pseudoparalysis (postneonatal Erb palsy)	
Leptomeningitis	
Ophthalmologic abnormalities	
Failure to thrive	

*Components of the Hutchinson triad.

■ Box 15–1
Surveillance Case Definition for
Congenital Syphilis

For reporting purposes, congenital syphilis includes cases of congenitally acquired syphilis in infants and children, as well as syphilitic stillbirths.

A confirmed case of congenital syphilis is an infant in whom *Treponema pallidum* is identified by dark-field microscopy, fluorescent antibody, or other specific stains in specimens from lesions, placenta, umbilical cord, or autopsy material.

A presumptive case of congenital syphilis is either of the following:

A. Any infant whose mother had untreated or inadequately treated syphilis at delivery (inadequate treatment consists of any nonpenicillin therapy or penicillin given <30 days prior to delivery), regardless of findings in the infant; or

B. Any infant or child who has a reactive treponemal test for syphilis and any one of the following:

   1. any evidence of congenital syphilis on physical examination (signs in an infant [<2 years of age] may include hepatosplenomegaly, characteristic skin rash, condyloma lata, snuffles, jaundice [syphilitic hepatitis], pseudo-paralysis, or edema [nephrotic syndrome]; stigmata in an older child may include interstitial keratitis, nerve deafness, anterior bowing of shins, frontal bossing, mulberry molars, Hutchinson's teeth, saddle nose, rhagades, or Clutton's joints); or

—— *continued* ——

■ **Box 15-1** (continued)

2. any evidence of congenital syphilis on long-bone radiograph; or

3. reactive cerebrospinal fluid (CSF) VDRL. It may be difficult to distinguish between congenital and acquired syphilis in a seropositive child after infancy. Signs may not be obvious, and stigmata may not yet have developed. Abnormal values for CSF VDRL, cell count, and protein, as well as IgM antibodies, may be found in either congenital or acquired syphilis. The decision may ultimately be based on maternal history and clinical judgment; the possibility of sexual abuse also needs to be considered; or

4. elevated CSF cell count or protein (without other cause); or

5. quantitative nontreponemal serologic titers that are fourfold higher than the mother's (both drawn at birth); or

6. reactive test for FTA ABS 19S-IgM antibody.

A syphilitic stillbirth is defined as a fetal death in which the mother had untreated or inadequately treated syphilis at delivery of a fetus after a 20-week gestation or of a fetus weighing >500 g.

From reference 17.

TABLE 15–5. EVALUATION FOR EARLY CONGENITAL SYPHILIS[19]

1. Maternal history, including results of serologic testing and treatment
2. Thorough physical examination
3. Long-bone radiographs
    A. Diaphyseal periostitis
    B. Osteochondritis
    C. Wimberger sign
4. Nontreponemal antibody titer
    A. VDRL test (simultaneous quantitative serum titer for mother and neonate)
5. Treponemal antibody titer
    A. FTA ABS test
    B. FTA ABS on 19S-IgM fraction of serum (CDC)
6. CSF analysis
    A. Cell count
    B. Protein level determination
    C. VDRL test
7. Other tests as clinically indicated
    A. Chest radiography
    B. Complete blood cell count
        1. Leukemoid reaction with or without monocytosis or lymphocytosis
        2. Coombs-negative hemolytic anemia
    C. Platelet count
        1. Thrombocytopenia
    D. Liver function tests
    E. Urinalysis
8. HIV antibody test

firmatory FTA ABS and IgM studies of FTA ABS, CSF analysis for cell count, protein level, and VDRL (Table 15–5). Other testing may be clinically indicated, and all infants should receive an antibody titer for HIV. Infants may also require extensive testing to confirm the HIV infection for the same reasons necessary for syphilis (ie, maternal antibodies).[19]

The newborn must be treated for probable neurosyphilis infection, and there may be difficulties in establishing this condition. See Fig. 15–1 for an algorithm for treatment. Each child should have a CSF evaluation done; the characteristic findings include a positive VDRL titer of the fluid, a mononuclear pleocytosis (5 to 100 cells/mm3), a moderately elevated protein level (30 to 75 mg/ml), and a normal glucose concentration. The CDC has recognized the difficulties in diagnosing neurosyphilis in infants with congenital syphilis and now recommends treatment with crystalline penicillin G or procaine penicillin G for a minimum of 10 days so as to also treat a CNS infection.[19]

This recommendation especially applies to infants who have no physical or laboratory evidence of congenital syphilis but who do have a positive HIV antibody test with antibodies from mother and/or infant. Each infant with HIV antibodies should have CSF analysis for neurosyphilis. These two sexually transmitted diseases share many of the same epidemiologic characteristics, but the concurrent HIV infection is thought to alter the manifestations of syphilis by impairing cell-mediated immunity to the syphilitic spirochete. The open chancre is thought to also enhance the introduction of HIV. The B-cell abnormalities associated with the HIV infection (hypergammaglobulinemia) may lead to unusually high VDRL titers.[19]

Treatment for the newborn with congenital syphilis must recognize the ambiguity in properly identifying infants who have neurosyphilis (Fig. 15–1). Some treatment failures have been reported with benzathine penicillin G, and this antibiotic does not establish levels in the CSF adequate to eradicate the spirochete. The CDC now recommends 100,000 to 150,000 units/kg per day IV of crystalline penicillin G or 50,000 units/kg per day IM of procaine penicillin G for 10 to 14 days.[19]

Difficulties in treating the infant's mother who has both an HIV infection and a syphilis infection may com-

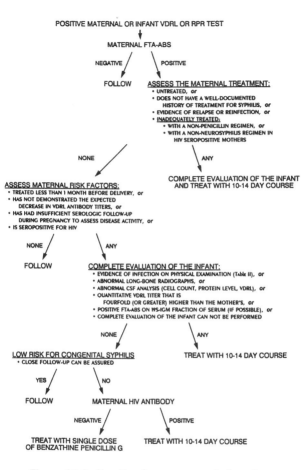

Figure 15–1. Algorithm for management of newborn infant born to mother with positive nontreponemal (VDRL or rapid plasma reagin) test result.[19]

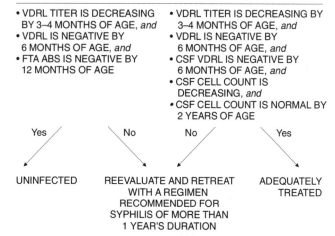

FOLLOW-UP FOR
UNTREATED INFANTS:
VDRL AND FTA ABS TITER
AT 1, 2, 4, 6, AND 12 MONTHS

FOLLOW-UP FOR
TREATED INFANTS:
VDRL TITER AT
1, 2, 4, 6, AND 12 MONTHS *and*
CSF ANALYSIS EVERY 6 MONTHS

• VDRL TITER IS DECREASING
  BY 3–4 MONTHS OF AGE, *and*
• VDRL IS NEGATIVE BY
  6 MONTHS OF AGE, *and*
• FTA ABS IS NEGATIVE BY
  12 MONTHS OF AGE

• VDRL TITER IS DECREASING BY
  3–4 MONTHS OF AGE, *and*
• VDRL IS NEGATIVE BY
  6 MONTHS OF AGE, *and*
• CSF VDRL IS NEGATIVE BY
  6 MONTHS OF AGE, *and*
• CSF CELL COUNT IS
  DECREASING, *and*
• CSF CELL COUNT IS NORMAL BY
  2 YEARS OF AGE

Yes / No   No / Yes

UNINFECTED   REEVALUATE AND RETREAT   ADEQUATELY
                 WITH A REGIMEN   TREATED
                 RECOMMENDED FOR
                 SYPHILIS OF MORE THAN
                 1 YEAR'S DURATION

Figure 15–2. Follow-up management for an infant examined or treated for congenital syphilis.[19]

promise treatment of the infant. Research has demonstrated that HIV-positive patients have a greater number of treatment failures in early syphilis for those given benzathine penicillin G, and this treatment will then not adequately eradicate the illness in the child.[19]

These difficulties with treatment make it imperative that all infants born to women with a positive reaction to syphilis be monitored closely (Fig. 15–2). Whether or not the infant had evidence of congenital syphilis, each child should be seen at 1, 2, 4, 6, and 12 months of age, and a VDRL titer should be done at each visit. For those infants born to a mother whose serum was VDRL positive but FTA ABS negative, the VDRL should be falling by 3 to

4 months of age and gone by 6 months of age. If not, the infant should be fully reexamined and treated. If the infant continues to have maternal FTA ABS antibodies beyond 1 year of age, that should be considered a treatment failure. Finally, if a mother develops secondary or tertiary syphilis after treatment for primary syphilis, her infant must be reevaluated.[19]

Those who have evidence of congenital syphilis should also be followed with VDRL titers. The titers should be nonreactive by 6 months. Infants with CSF abnormalities should be followed every 6 months until the fluid is normal. If the CSF VDRL is positive at 6 months, the infant should be treated again. In addition, the CSF abnormalities should be returning to normal at each examination. If not, or if the CSF cell count is abnormal at 2 years of age, the infant should be treated again. The child should also be followed for evidence of neurologic or ophthalmologic abnormalities associated with syphilis.[19]

■ Prophylaxis for PCP

As in adults, PCP is the most common AIDS-associated condition in children, but they are less able to cope with infection. In cases reported to the CDC, 35% of children with PCP died within 2 months of their diagnosis. The CDC released recommendations for prophylaxis of children based on experience with other immunocompromising conditions in children.[20] Trimethoprim-sulfamethoxazole (TMP-SMX) at a dose of 150 mg/m^2 TMP and 750 mg/m^2 SMX in divided doses either daily or three consecutive days per week is effective in preventing PCP. See Table 15–6 for therapy alternatives. The following guidelines for T4 counts indicate when TMP-SMX should be initiated:

- < 1500 for children 1 to 11 months
- < 750 for children 12 to 23 months

TABLE 15–6. DRUG REGIMENS FOR PCP PROPHYLAXIS[5]

Recommended Regimen (children ≥1 month of age):
Trimethoprim/sulfamethoxazole (TMP-SMX) 150 mg
TMP/m^2/day with 750 mg SMX/m^2/day given orally in divided
doses twice a day (b.i.d.) 3 times per week on consecutive
days (eg, Monday-Tuesday-Wednesday)

Acceptable alternative TMP-SMX dosage schedules:

A. 150 mg TMP/m^2/day with 750 mg SMX/m^2/day given orally
as a single daily dose 3 times per week on consecutive
days (eg, M-T-W)

B. 150 mg TMP/m^2/day with 750 mg SMX/m^2/day orally divided
b.i.d. and **given 7 days/week**

C. 150 mg TMP/m^2/day with 750 mg SMX/m^2/day given orally
divided b.i.d. and given 3 times per week on **alternate days**
(eg, M-W-F)

Alternative Regimens, if TMP-SMX Not Tolerated:
Aerosolized pentamidine (≥5 years of age) 300 mg given via
Respirgard II inhaler monthly.

Dapsone (≥1 month of age) 1 mg/kg (not to exceed 100 mg)
given orally once daily.

If neither aerosolized pentamidine nor dapsone is tolerated,
some clinicians use **intravenous pentamidine** (4 mg/kg)
given every 2 or 4 weeks.

- < 500 for children 24 months through 5 years
- < 200 for children 6 years and older

A T4 percentage of 20% or less also warrants prophylaxis for PCP.[20]

■ Zidovudine Treatment for Children

Zidovudine (ZDV or AZT) has not been studied as extensively in children as in adults, though clinical trials do demonstrate an improvement in the child's condition while receiving the medication. In a recent review of clinical trials of zidovudine,[21] improvements were noted in neurodevelopmental abnormalities, cognitive abilities, appetite and weight gain, as well as decreased lymph node and liver size, decreased immunoglobulin values, and increased T4 cell counts. Oral zidovudine also brought about reductions in p24 antigen levels in CSF as well as reversal of the CSF cultures for HIV for most of the children (6 of 7) who were enrolled in a recent clinical trial. This results in improvement in neuropsychological activity, even when the most common AIDS-indicator disease in this clinical trial was encephalopathy. These studies evaluated children from infancy to preteens, and different dosages, both oral and intravenous, were used. As in adults, higher levels resulted in anemia and neutropenia for a significant number of children. The usual oral dosage for these clinical trials was 180 mg/m^2 every 6 hours or four times a day. The best dosage for infected children must still be determined.[22] Other side effects from ZDV include nausea, myalgia, insomnia, and severe headaches.[23]

■ Immunizations for HIV-Positive Children

Children with the HIV infection are at high risk for fulminant cases of childhood illnesses, including a fatal outcome from measles and chickenpox.[3] Hence, immunizations become more important and should be carefully considered when treating patients[24] (Table 15–7).

■ Periodic Evaluation of Infants Born to HIV-Positive Mothers

Table 15–8 summarizes the evaluation of an infant born to an HIV-positive mother.[22]

■ Psychosocial Aspects of HIV in Children and Adolescents

Children with HIV/AIDS frequently have developmental delays and progressive loss of cognitive function.

TABLE 15–7. IMMUNIZATIONS FOR THE CHILD WITH HIV/AIDS[24]

Vaccine	Known asymptomatic	Symptomatic
DPT	Yes	Yes
OPV	No	No
IPV	Yes	Yes
MMR	Yes	Yes
Hibc	Yes	Yes
Pneumococcal*	No	Yes
Influenza*	No	Yes

Please note that inactivated polio (IPV) is given, but children continue to receive live MMR vaccines. There has been little vaccine-associated illness with the measles vaccine, but the risk of severe measles is great in children with AIDS.[22]
*Pneumococcal vaccine should be given at age 2 years. The influenza vaccine should be given yearly starting at age 6 months.
Used with permission of the American Academy of Pediatrics.

Delays are most common in fine and gross motor skills as well as speech. These may be directly related to CNS infection with HIV. Manifestations of infection include microcephaly and radiographic evidence of cerebral atrophy. School-age children also perform poorly when undergoing testing for intelligence.[25]

Children are also at risk for depression because they have a chronic disease that presently is universally fatal. Common symptoms include apathy, withdrawal, and anorexia. Children and adolescents may also develop dementia and psychosis. Little has been done to study these conditions directly in children and adolescents, but they have been observed to have similar symptoms to adults with AIDS who suffer from AIDS dementia or encephalopathy. Treatment includes rehabilitation, psychopharmacology, and psychotherapy.[25] Some unique aspects of pediatric HIV disease are found in Table 15–9.

TABLE 15–8. RECOMMENDED FOLLOW-UP SCHEDULE FOR ASYMPTOMATIC INFANTS BORN TO HIV-SEROPOSITIVE MOTHERS: A CONSENSUS OPINION OF PEDIATRIC INFECTIOUS DISEASES TRAINING PROGRAM DIRECTORS

Evaluations	No. of Times Performed during the First Year of Life	Ages (months) That We Would Recommend for Evaluations	No. of Times Performed during the Second Year of Life	Ages (months) That We Would Recommend for Evaluations
History and physical examination	3–12	0, 3, 6, 9, 12	2–5	15, 18, 21, 24
Neurodevelopmental testing	0–12	6, 12	1–4	24
Complete blood count and platelet count	1–6	0, 3, 6, 9, 12	0–4	15, 18, 21, 24
Renal function tests	0–5	0, 6, 12	0–4	18, 24
Liver function tests	0–5	0, 6, 12	0–4	18, 24
Serum immunoglobulins	0–6	6, 12	0–4	24
Lymphocyte subsets	0–6	0, 3, 6, 9, 12	0–4	15, 18, 21, 24
Lymphocyte proliferation assays	0–4	NR	0–3	NR
HIV antibody (enzyme-linked immunosorbent assay)	0–6	0, 3, 6, 9, 12	1–4	15, 18, 21, 24
HIV antibody (Western blot)	0–6	if + ELISA	0–4	15, 18, 21, 24
HIV p24 antigen assay	0–6	0, 3, 6, 9, 12	0–4	15, 18, 21, 24
HIV peripheral blood culture	0–5	0, 3, 6, 9, 12	0–4	15, 18, 21, 24
HIV PCR assay	0–5	0, 3, 6, 9, 12	0–4	15, 18, 21, 24
Lumbar puncture	0–1	12	0–1	24
Electroencephalograph	0–2	12	0–2	24
Chest radiograph	0–2	12	0–2	24
Head computed axial tomographic scan and/or magnetic resonance imaging	0–1	12	0–1	24
Electrocardiography/ECHO	0–2	12	0–2	24

NR, not recommended.
From reference 22: Prober CG, Gershon AA. Medical management of newborns and infants born to human immunodeficiency virus-seropositive mothers. *Pediatr Infect Dis J.* 1991;10:684–695. Copyright © Williams & Wilkins, 1991.

TABLE 15-9. UNIQUE ASPECTS OF PEDIATRIC HIV DISEASE[26]

The almost invariable illness of the biologic mother, and often other family members

The preponderance of cases among minority families, including some from Third World countries with endemic infection

The association of the infection with drug use and poverty

The frequent provision of care by persons other than the parents (foster parents, extended family, institutions)

The uncertainty in establishing the diagnosis in the newborn

Its nature as an infectious disease

The special stigma and potential hysteria surrounding AIDS, and the consequent extraordinary need for confidentiality

The rapidity of advance in clinical knowledge and the need to disseminate these advances promptly to affected families

The geographic clustering of cases

The intensity of services needed to maintain optimal health and family function

The disproportionate reliance on public financing and health care institutions for medical care

The dramatic potential for prevention

References

1. Centers for Disease Control and Prevention. *HIV/AIDS Surveillance Report.* October, 1992;1–18.

2. Caldwell MB, Rogers MF. Epidemiology of the pediatric AIDS infection. In: Edelson PJ, ed. Childhood AIDS. *Pediatr Clin North Am.* 1991;38:1–16.

3. Burroughs MB, Edelson PJ. Medical care of the HIV-infected child. In: Edelson PJ, ed. Childhood AIDS. *Pediatr Clin North Am.* 1991;38:45–68.

4. Centers for Disease Control. Classification system for human immunodeficiency virus (HIV) infection in children under 13 years of age. *MMWR.* 1987;36(15):225–236.

5. Centers for Disease Control. Guidelines for prophylaxis against *Pneumocystis carinii* pneumonia for chil-

dren infected with the human immunodeficiency virus. *MMWR.* 1991;40(RR-2):1–13.

6. European Collaborative Study. Children born to women with HIV-1 infection: natural history and risk of infection. *Lancet.* 1991;337:253–260.

7. American Academy of Pediatrics, Task Force on Pediatric AIDS. Perinatal human immunodeficiency virus (HIV) testing. *AAP News.* 1992;8:20–25.

8. Rogers MF, Chin-Yin O, Kilborne B, Schochetman G. Advances and problems in the diagnosis of human immunodeficiency virus infection in infants. *Pediatr Infect Dis J.* 1991:10:523–531.

9. Weiblen BJ, Lee FK, Cooper ER, et al. Early diagnosis of HIV infections in infants by detection of IgA antibodies. *Lancet.* 1990;335:988–990.

10. Centers for Disease Control and Prevention. *HIV/Aids Surveillance Report.* February, 1993;1–18.

11. Sanders-Laufer D, DeBruin W, Edelson PJ. *Pneumocystis carinii* infections in HIV-infected children. In: Edelson PJ, ed. Childhood AIDS. *Pediatr Clin North Am.* 1991;38:69–88.

12. Pitt J. Lymphocytic interstitial pneumonia. In: Edelson PJ, ed. Childhood AIDS. *Pediatr Clin North Am.* 1991;38:89–95.

13. Braun MM, Cauthen G. Relationship of the human immunodeficiency virus epidemic to pediatric tuberculosis and *Bacillus Calmette-Guerin* immunization. *Pediatr Infect Dis J.* 1992;11:220–227.

14. American Thoracic Society and the Centers for Disease Control. Diagnostic standards and classification of tuberculosis. *Am Rev Respir Dis.* 1990;142:725–735.

15. Starke JR. Modern approach to the diagnosis and management of tuberculosis in children. In: Kaplan SL, ed. *Pediatr Clin North Am.* 1988;35:441–464.

16. Kuzal RJ, Clutter DJ. Current perspectives on respiratory syncytial virus infections. *Postgrad Med.* 1993;93: 129–141.

17. Centers for Disease Control. Congenital syphilis—New York City, 1986–1988. *MMWR.* 1989;38(48):825–829.

18. Zenker PN, Rolfs RT. Treatment of syphilis, 1989. *Rev Infect Dis.* 1990;12(supp 6):S590–S609.

19. Ikeda MK, Jenson HB. Evaluation and treatment of congenital syphilis. *J Pediatr.* 1990;117(6):843–852.

20. Centers for Disease Control. Guidelines for prophylaxis against *Pneumocystis carinii* pneumonia for children infected with human immunodeficiency virus. *MMWR.* 1991;40(RR-2):1–13.

21. McKinney RE Jr., Maha MA, Conner EM, et al. A multicenter trial of oral zidovudine in children with advanced human immunodeficiency virus disease. *N Engl J Med.* 1991;324:1018–1025.

22. Prober CG, Gershon AA. Medical management of newborns and infants born to human immunodeficiency virus-seropositive mothers. *Pediatr Infect Dis J.* 1991;10:684–695.

23. Richmond DD, Fischl MA, Grieco MH, et al. The toxicity of azidothymidine (AZT) in the treatment of patients with AIDS and AIDS-related complex: A double-blind, placebo controlled trial. *N Engl J Med.* 1987;317:192–197.

24. Committee on Infectious Disease, American Academy of Pediatrics and The Centers for Disease Control. *Report of the committee on infectious disease,* 22nd ed. Elk Grove Village, IL: American Academy of Pediatrics; 1991.

25. Speigal L, Mayars A. Psychological aspects of AIDS in children and adolescents. In: Edelson PJ, ed. Childhood AIDS. *Pediatr Clin North Am.* 1988;35:441–464.

26. Meyers A, Weitzman M. Pediatric HIV disease: The newest chronic illness of childhood. In: Edelson PJ, ed. Childhood AIDS. *Pediatr Clin North Am.* 1991;38:169–194.

Chapter Sixteen

SOCIAL WORKER ASSESSMENT AND INTERVENTION

MIGUEL A. ORTEGA, MSW, ACSW, CSW-ACP

The role of the social worker in the treatment of those affected by HIV is multifaceted. Social worker practice consists of professional interventions that enhance the development, problem-solving, and coping capacities of people. The profession promotes the effective and humane operation of medical, social, and educational systems that link people to resources and services, educates them about how to better utilize them, and contributes to the development and improvement of social policies and programs.[1] In the medical setting, social workers are involved in evaluation of patients' coping abilities, support network, resource systems, and their basic needs including financial, emotional, employment, and adjustment.

The initial evaluation done by a social worker is a complete psychosocial history that may include a personal history, family history, dynamics of relationships, educational and employment history, understanding of medical situation, past and present coping strategies and mechanisms employed, and resources presently being used to meet needs. With this information the professional social worker should assess:

1. level of understanding the HIV-positive individual has of his or her medical condition;
2. make-up and dynamics of personal support system and networks;
3. past coping mechanisms with focus on what is needed to handle present situation;
4. level of financial security and resource needs; and
5. advocacy and educational needs within medical resource systems.

This evaluation, combined with the social worker's knowledge about the roles and duties of the other professionals (ie, physicians, nurses, physician assistants, and rehabilitation specialists) involved, allows the social worker to provide direct interventions such as counseling, medical regimen education, advocacy, and referral. The social worker also provides consultative services to the other members of the team regarding the special needs or social circumstances of the individual patient, family, or significant others. This service includes being information brokers of current programs and the eligibility criteria for each program. In order to expand on the chapter regarding psychosocial issues (Chapter 21), this chapter focuses on how to evaluate the impact of those issues on the HIV-positive patient, as well as specific interventions and resource tips.

■ Evaluation of the Person Who Is HIV Positive or Has AIDS

Identifying the diagnosis (HIV/AIDS) and whether it is a new diagnosis for the patient will help establish the potential need for crisis intervention. Although we all cope differently, the social worker needs to be prepared for dealing with an emotionally devastated individual. Determining the extent of the patient's knowledge and understanding of the diagnosis allows for the identification of:

1. continued educational needs regarding health status and assistance with reframing of perspectives;
2. communication and assertiveness skills needed to enhance patients' abilities to become a partner in their own care; and
3. the need for "safer sex" counseling and education.

Determining the patient's current emotional state requires the social worker to investigate the presence of denial, anger, guilt, hopelessness, or other signs of clinical depression, including suicide risk factors. This allows for identifying and supporting the emotional well-being of the patient. Because of its severity, special attention is given to suicide risk. Individuals are considered to be at risk for suicide and in need of an evaluation if they have:

1. a noted past history of suicidal ideations or attempts, impulse control problems, known clinical depression, substance abuse, and/or a psychiatric diagnosis;
2. experienced an increase in personal losses in the past 6 months with significant impact including deaths, loss of financial support, and/or loss of physical and mental capacities;
3. changes in sleep, eating, social, or recreation habits that are found to be inhibiting their ability to function;
4. coping patterns that are inappropriate, such as substance abuse or violence; or
5. made direct statements regarding a desire to die or give up.

If the patient is thought to be at risk, special attention needs to be given to evaluating the patient's support network, coping skills, changes in behavior, hygiene, and emotional status. If the patient states that suicide is the intent, then the worker needs to assess:

1. the difference between ideation, threats, and gestures;
2. lethality of the means chosen and availability;
3. detail of plan;
4. preparation (ie, developing wills, giving away belongings);
5. desire and ability; and
6. intent to live or die.

The preceding information will be helpful with the intervention of the suicidal patient.

The evaluation of the social support system and basic needs (Table 16–1) of the patient includes identification of pertinent persons making up the system, their roles, how they see themselves in this system, and the strengths and weaknesses of the system itself. This may include strong

TABLE 16–1. EVALUATION OF BASIC NEEDS

Living arrangements
Financial situation
Medical situation
Transportation
Activities of daily living

Note: A patient's own perceptions of his or her physical functioning compared to the social worker's observations gives insight into self-image and denial. This should also be based on the findings of the occupational and physical therapists as well as work evaluations for the purpose of career counseling or adaptation to working with disabilities. A referral to the state vocational and rehabilitation agency and counseling regarding awareness of rights guaranteed under the Americans with Disabilities Act should be considered.

family ties or friendships that may impact physical and emotional health. Obtaining a good understanding of the openness of communication related to the disease identifies individuals who may be experiencing denial, rejection, isolation, a need for counseling regarding partner notification, or a mechanism to vent fears. The ability of the support system to meet the patient's needs will identify the need for referrals to agencies and programs to help meet those needs. If community agencies are already involved, this knowledge indicates the individual's ability to use available resources appropriately.

Behaviors that impact on the patient's health and/or medical treatment need to be identified and assessed. These include, but are not limited to, IDU, other substance use, unprotected high-risk sexual practices, and noncompliance with medical regimens. This information is useful to the medical team and identifies possible obstacles and challenges in assisting the individual to address those goals and needs.

The final part of the assessment should include a discussion of the direction the patient wants to take from this point on regarding treatment and other life issues. The social worker should allow the patient to prioritize the identified needs. It is important to note that because of time constraints involved in doing a thorough assessment, the patient's identified needs and concerns may be all that are dealt with in the initial interview. The larger assessment may need to be done in a second, scheduled interview.

■ Interventions

Patient education about the HIV/AIDS disease process, with an information packet specific to the patient's situation (ie, stage of illness, social situation, and language and cultural consideration) is necessary. This provides written reinforcement to verbal education. It allows individuals to educate themselves at a pace with which they can cope, and provide them with materials to begin to educate family and loved ones.

Interventions for patients in denial about their diagnosis or risk groups may also help with the acceptance of the diagnosis and enhance transmission precautions. The first step is education, followed by continual reinforcement of the realities of early intervention and treatment. Open discussions about their diagnosis and the possibility of rejection and death can lead to acknowledgment. In order to establish trust, an open atmosphere with nonjudgmental materials and staff is essential.

Patient empowerment of self-advocacy gives individuals control over their own lives. This empowerment makes coping easier when feelings of hopelessness exist or if the terminal nature of the disease is the issue. Basic topics to cover with patients include taking personal responsibility for their own medical treatment, nutrition, exercise, and stress reduction. Interventions could include educational pamphlets, seminars, assertiveness skill training, meditation, religion, and spiritual healing.

Discussion of issues relating to large, bureaucratic clinics or hospital systems can maximize the appropriate utilization of the available health care services. It can also increase the ability to cope with large and continuously changing teaching and health care institutions and understanding how health care systems function.

Grief counseling for losses such as the death of loved ones from AIDS, finances, professional identity, physical functioning, appearance, independence, control of life, social support, and family support is an important skill in the social worker repertoire. Interventions may include crisis intervention techniques to allow for controlled venting of emotions, referral to various agencies and programs to address financial and career losses, and referrals to support groups for ongoing assistance to deal with the loss or losses.

Some individuals faced with HIV/AIDS may have feelings of guilt that can be related to the possibility of spreading the disease, unresolved identity issues, survivor's guilt, or lack of independence.

The resolution of guilt can be facilitated by allowing individuals to express their feelings in a supportive environment. Patients should consider specialized therapy or support group involvement, as well as plan for the possibility of dependence and discuss what things can be done to prolong activity, control, and remain independent mentally with physical limitations.

If the patient is a substance abuser and acknowledges that use or abuse is a problem that needs addressing, a referral to an appropriate substance abuse program is indicated. If the patient is in denial concerning substance usage, the intervention should be to reinforce the clinician's concerns about the effects of substance use on the disease and the treatment. Although change is not possible unless the patient is willing to verbalize a problem, attempts to educate the patient should continue.

Counseling patients on the disclosure of the diagnosis to family, friends, and employer involves decision counseling. To start, help the individual ascertain why disclosure is necessary at this time. Is it work related? A need for support? Out of fear or uncertainty? Pamphlets or other written materials on this topic may be helpful to the patient. This will give the patient basic information and steps in identifying to whom, when, where, and how to disclose this information. The decision should be planned and not a single-session decision.

It is imperative that all health care professionals be able to manage the suicidal patient. Suicide ideations, gestures, or threats that occur during telephone follow-up

■ Box 16-1
Steps in the Management of the Suicidal Patient

1. Make someone aware that you are handling a suicide and have a trace placed on the call if notified by telephone.
2. Notify the mental health authorities.
3. Ask the patient to delay the suicide plan.
4. Check for detail of plan, availability and lethality of plan, and desire to die.
5. Assess whether substances have already been used such as alcohol or cannabis that may further impair the patient's ability to reason.
6. If a telephone contact, check to see if the patient is alone or if others are at the patient's location.
7. Help the patient identify the level and sources of stress.
8. Actively help the patient review options to solve current problem.
9. Use the patient's personal resources and your professional resources to try and resolve the most pressing issues.
10. Contract with the patient not to proceed with the suicide plan for a set period of time and to follow through with the resource plan. Be certain that the patient is able to be realistic.
11. If a phone trace is possible, keep client on the telephone line until the mental health authorities arrive.
12. Refer for appropriate psychiatric evaluation.

■ **Box 16–2**
Long-Term Management Issues in
Suicide

1. If the patient is suicidal, inform the patient's clinician of the suicide risk and refer to an appropriate psychiatric service, such as a crisis clinic, or consult psychiatry.
2. If the patient is clinically depressed, inform the patient's clinician and request psychiatric consultation. Follow the patient to reinforce the psychiatric plan and offer case management services.
3. If the patient is undergoing multiple stressors, help the patient identify issues and begin a plan to deal with each one. Refer the patient to a support group for HIV-positive persons and follow up weekly by phone and in clinic with regard to follow-through with referrals, plans made in counseling sessions, and emotional status.

calls should be treated as real. A crisis intervention technique should be used (Boxes 16–1 and 16–2).

■ Community Resources

The following is a list of various national resources that may be helpful in identifying resources for patients. It is important to identify those agencies that are in close proximity to the patient. Most local AIDS organizations offer support in counseling, food, equipment loans, housing, minimal financial assistance, transportation, in-home nursing care, and buddy programs.

- National AIDS Hotline
  800-342-AIDS
- CDC National Sexually Transmitted Diseases Hotline
  800-227-8922
- Center for Substance Abuse Treatment (CSAT)
  800-662-HELP
- Hospice Link
  800-331-1620
- Gay Men's Health Crisis
  212-807-6655
- National AIDS Clearinghouse
  800-458-5231
- Clinical Trials
  800-TRIALS-A

Reference

1. National Association of Social Workers. A Definition of Social Work Practice. *NASW Standards for the Classification of Social Work Practice—Policy Statement IV.* 1981:6.

....
....
....
....

Chapter Seventeen

Dentistry and AIDS

T.C. Lyon, Jr., DDS, PhD

No other disease in history has so dramatically altered the practice of dentistry as has AIDS. It has resulted in the institution of stringent disinfection and sterilization procedures monitored by OSHA, and only now being carried over to medicine. It has raised medical-legal as well as ethical and moral issues that have resulted in the loss to the profession of trained ancillary as well as other office personnel and in the decision of some practitioners to leave the profession. Recognition of the inevitable mortality of this disease has resulted in the presentation of many well-attended continuing education courses related to all aspects of the disease including prevention, diagnosis, and treatment. This interest is heightened by the facts that a health-conscious population will visit the dental office more frequently than that of other health care providers, resulting in contact with patients who may or may not be aware of their infection, and the oral cavity may show some of the first manifestations of the disease. A wide range of conditions may show oral manifestations associated with HIV infection. Table 17–1 lists a number of these conditions.

TABLE 17–1. ORAL MANIFESTATIONS ASSOCIATED WITH HIV INFECTION

Bacterial Infections

Actinomycosis
Cat scratch disease
Submandibular cellulitis
HIV-necrotizing gingivitis
HIV-gingivitis
HIV-periodontitis

Infections caused by the following oral opportunistic pathogens:

Mycobacterium avium intracellulare
Klebsiella pneumoniae
Enterobacterium cloacae
Escherichia coli

Viral Infections

Herpes simplex virus
Cytomegalovirus
Epstein-Barr virus
  Hairy leukoplakia
Varicella-zoster virus diseases
Herpes zoster
Varicella
Human papilloma virus diseases
  Verruca vulgaris
  Condyloma acuminatum
  Focal epithelial hyperplasia

Fungal Infections

Candidiasis
  Pseudomembranous
  Erythematous
  Hyperplastic
  Angular cheilitis
Histoplasmosis
Cryptococcoses
Geotrichosis

Neoplasms

Kaposi's sarcoma
Squamous cell carcinoma
Non-Hodgkin's lymphoma

Neurologic Disturbances

Trigeminal neuropathy
Facial palsy

Unknown Etiology

Recurrent aphthous stomatitis
Salivary gland enlargement
Xerostomia
Delayed wound healing
Major aphthae

Note: This list is not all-inclusive.

Although information is available on all the conditions listed in Table 17–1, further discussion is provided on the following: oral candidiasis, hairy leukoplakia, oral recurrent herpes simplex, and HIV gingivitis, HIV necrotizing gingivitis, and HIV periodontitis.

■ Oral Candidiasis

This is considered to be the most common oral infection in HIV patients and may frequently be diagnosed prior to recognition of HIV infection. It may be manifested in a number of ways:

1. Simple angular cheilitis.
2. Angular cheilitis and "hairy leukoplakia" of the tongue.
3. The classical pseudomembranous form, which may be limited to the palate, buccal mucosa, or tongue, or may involve all surfaces.
4. An atrophic form, which may show generalized inflammation with few white lesions, or be telangiectatic (ie, many petite hemorrhagic areas on the palate).
5. Lesions of the tongue which may resemble migratory glossitis.
6. Burning of the tongue or pain involving the palate.

■ Hairy Leukoplakia

This condition was first noted in 1981 and is now included in the CDC classification and is recognized as a common feature of HIV. It may even be more common than oral candidiasis. The lesion usually appears as a white patch on the lateral border or borders of the tongue. It rarely occurs on the mucosa of the cheeks, the floor of the mouth, the soft palate, or the oropharynx. The irregular surface of the lesion may appear as projections that resemble hairs, hence the name. It is usually asymptomatic but may become superinfected with *Candida.* It is fairly accurate as an indicator of infection with HIV and tends to indicate a reduced immunocompetence. It must be differentiated from a number of other white oral lesions.

■ Oral Recurrent Herpes Simplex

Recurrent herpes labialis (cold sores) are frequently seen in the general population; however, they are more frequently seen among individuals infected with HIV than among noninfected individuals. Further, these lesions recur more frequently, are larger, and may persist. In fact, in an HIV-infected individual, if the lesions last for more than 1 month, they meet the CDC definition of AIDS.

Recurrent intraoral HSV infection may also be seen. Again, the lesions recur more frequently and persist longer. Although they appear more frequently on the hard palate and attached gingiva, they may be found on any mucosal surface.

■ HIV Gingivitis, HIV Necrotizing Gingivitis, and HIV Periodontitis

It is well recognized that young adult male AIDS patients show a higher than expected frequency of periodontal problems. These lesions of the gingiva and periodontium are unusual and exhibit the following clinical characteristics:

1. Pain or discomfort.
2. A gingivitis that may show necrosis and/or inflammation.
3. Rapid and progressive gingival recession and bone loss.
4. Alveolar bone loss.

These symptoms appear to correlate with loss of immunocompetence.

Chapter Eighteen

NURSING ASSESSMENT OF HIV-POSITIVE PATIENTS

BARBARA CARNES, RN, CS, PhD
JANICE POUNDS, RN

Because of the chronic nature of HIV infection, the professional relationship between the patient and the health care worker is likely to be a long-term one. The American Nurses Association (ANA) suggests that long-term care can be defined as the "provision of the range of services—physical, psychological, spiritual, social, and economic—all that is needed to help people attain, maintain, or regain their optimum level of functioning."[1] Additionally, the ANA proposes that this definition include any person or group needing health care over an extended period. Based in a holistic framework and with a broad knowledge base, nurses are in a unique position to have a profound impact on the patient's response to HIV infection over time.

Since HIV can affect any body system, thorough assessment and analysis of the physical, psychological, spiritual, social, and economic impact of HIV, in collaboration with the patient, can lead to the accurate identification of actual or potential problems and contributing factors that are amenable to nursing intervention. It is our hope that this chapter will reinforce previous knowledge and enable nurses to enhance their skills in assessing the impact of HIV on the individual. Since nursing interventions address the nursing diagnosis rather than a specific medical diagnosis, nurses will discover that creative application of existing nursing interventions will be quite appropriate when working with this clientele.

■ Self-Assessment

Working with individuals who are HIV-positive can bring nurses into contact with those whose lifestyles are different from or run parallel to their own. In the former case, the nurse might be tempted to criticize them; in the latter case, the situation may stir up unresolved past conflicts in the nurse. The potential for development of an effective nurse/patient relationship is jeopardized in either case. It is important to remember that communication is a two-way process; just as nurses are attuned to their patients' verbal and non-verbal messages, patients are also sensitive to the message sent by their nurses. Therefore, prior to assessing other individuals, it is imperative that nurses and other health care providers examine their own beliefs, values, and feelings associated with sexuality, alternative lifestyles, drug use, and family dysfunction, including abuse and infidelity. Personal concerns related to all of these areas, as well as to death and dying, can be transmitted consciously or unconsciously to the patient and can interfere with the nurses' ability to collaborate effectively with individuals who are HIV-positive.

■ Communication

Effective communication skills are fundamental to the nursing process. Attention to communication during the initial assessment phase can provide the foundation for a therapeutic relationship between the patient and the nurse. The effective use of communication techniques such as listening, open-ended questions, focused question, clarifying, and paraphrasing will not only elicit information but will also communicate caring, concern, and respect for the patient (Box 18–1).

■ Box 18–1
Selected Communication Techniques[2,3]

- *Listening:* Actively attends to patient's verbal and nonverbal behavior in order to comprehend the patient's message.
- *Open-ended question:* Provides patients with the opportunity to respond to question in their own words (eg, "Tell me about your week").
- *Focused question:* Provides patient with the opportunity to respond to question in their own words while limiting the scope of the question (eg, "Tell me about your appetite since your last clinic visit").
- *Paraphrasing:* Uses own words to communicate to patient the content (restating) or the feeling (reflection) message heard by the nurse.
- *Clarifying:* Asks for more information in order to understand patient message.
- *Validating:* Uses own words to restate or reflect message to verify accuracy.

Although AIDS is often described as a disease of loss, it is clear that in some cases HIV infection may provide an opportunity for personal growth and self-actualization. Some patients have reported that after an initial period of adjusting to the reality of being HIV-positive, they have noticed a positive change in the way in which they live. They express an increased inner peace and satisfaction in living. Hymovich and Hagopian[4] assert that "not everyone exposed to a stressor will have adverse health effects. . . . stress may enhance growth and development under some circumstances" (140–141).

In order to gain insight into the patient's perspective, it is helpful to ask questions such as "What do you understand about your condition?" and "What does being HIV-positive mean to you?" The patient's answers to questions such as these provide the nurse with the opportunity to correct misconceptions and to provide information about resources that are available to the patient. At these times, it is important to introduce the idea that individuals do have control over the way they respond to the disease and the way they choose to take care of themselves.

Assessment is an ongoing process. Careful initial assessment facilitates the identification of current problems and also provides a baseline from which the nurse can identify subtle changes over time. A solid data base is the foundation on which nurses build the framework of interventions focused on actual and potential responses that impact the individual's well-being and quality of life. It might take several sessions to complete this initial assessment. Throughout the assessment process it is also important to identify the patient's unique strengths and talents that can be fostered or reinforced throughout the nurse/patient relationship. The therapeutic relationship between the nurse and patient begins with the first contact and the assessment process.

■ Patient Assessment

In reality, it is effective to be alert to all aspects of the individual throughout the assessment process. Physical health is impacted by psychosocial stressors just as psychological wellness is affected by physical health.

Anxiety

Throughout the interaction the nurse must be alert to the patient's level of anxiety. Clues to the patient's level of anxiety can be found in both verbal and nonverbal messages. Accurate assessment is important because it enables the nurse to tailor subsequent communication approaches to match the individual's need.[5] For example, when an individual is in a mild to moderate level of anxiety, it is likely that the assessment process will include several levels of problem solving and could include discussion of past, current, and future actions, thoughts, and feelings.[6] On the other hand, when the nurse identifies physiological, cognitive, behavioral, and/or emotional indicators of increasing anxiety, then the nurse would acknowledge the discomfort of the patient and note, for further exploration, the content areas that contribute to an increase in the severity of anxiety. The nurse returns to the assessment process and employs strategies that would require a lower degree of cognitive task and an easier level of communication, such as asking for a description of present or recent past actions and thoughts.

However, if the anxiety-producing issue relates to patient safety (ie, thoughts of suicide), it is imperative that the area be addressed when presented. Many individuals view a positive HIV test as equivalent to an AIDS diagnosis and often respond as if they have received a death sentence. It is essential that the nurse be alert to indications that the patient might intend to harm him- or herself or others. If such indicators are present, asking questions

■ Box 18-2
Suicide Assessment[7,8]

Evaluate Suicide Risk
1. Is there a history of previous suicide attempts?
2. Does content of message relate to death, suicide, wanting to be dead, wanting to spare others suffering?
3. Does patient fear nighttime or fear inability to sleep?
4. Has there been a change in sleep patterns?
5. Is mood depressed, worried, tense, hopeless, helpless?
6. Has there been a sudden increase in the patient's mood?
7. Does the patient seem driven to settle affairs?
8. Does the patient have a pattern of impulsive behavior?

Evaluate intent: "Are you thinking about harming yourself?"
1. If yes, then ask: "Do you have a plan?"
2. If yes, then state: "Tell me what you plan to do."

Evaluate plan: Is it lethal?
1. Does the patient have access to the means including the energy to carry out the plan?
2. Is there a chance for discovery and rescue by others?

about suicidal intent does not increase the risk of suicide. On the contrary, a question such as, "You seem to be having a very difficult time right now, are you thinking about hurting yourself?" brings the topic out in the open and provides the patient an opportunity to talk about concerns (Box 18–2). If necessary, consultation with other members of the health care team and referral of the patient to psychiatric/mental health specialists is helpful. Refer to Chapter 16 for further discussion on suicide interventions.

Physical Assessment

Physical assessment of the HIV-infected patient is discussed in Chapter 14.

Psychosocial Assessment

It is helpful to inquire into the patient's current concerns, fears, and expectations. Each patient is unique, and issues that cause concern for one might not cause concern for another. At times during the relationship, it is not unusual for individuals to have concerns about issues unrelated to HIV infection. For example, one patient expressed concern that people would not believe him when he denied that his sadness was related to his HIV status. He stated that his grandmother, who had been very loving to him, had died recently and that he felt very sad about this loss. It is helpful that nurses be alert to any area of patient concern and that they be willing to promote activities that help the individual deal with the stress.

It is important to help the patient identify current and previous methods for dealing with stress, the effectiveness of the methods used, and whether or not the patient is motivated to explore new ways of dealing with the stress. For some individuals, HIV infection is the first crisis with which they have had to deal.

Grief Stages

As stated earlier, some patients receive the news that they are HIV-positive as though it were a death sentence. This, as well as other losses encountered while living with HIV, can trigger the grief process, and it is common for some clients to go through some or all of the stages of grief that Dr. Elisabeth Kübler-Ross has identified[9,10] (Table 18–1). These stages are: (1) denial, (2) bargaining, (3) anger, (4) depression, and (5) acceptance. This is not to say that all individuals experience all stages or to say that the stages proceed in any given order. In fact, it is not unusual for patients to reach acceptance of their HIV status and

TABLE 18–1. STAGES OF GRIEF AND ASSOCIATED BEHAVIORS[9–12]

Denial
Allows individual time to process information and activate defenses (eg, fails to believe diagnosis and seeks multiple opinions from clinicians, unwilling to acknowledge symptoms, continues routine behavior).

Anger
Reaction to unfinished business, unfulfilled wishes (eg, feels that nothing is right. Anger, hostility, and high-risk behavior are common).

Bargaining
Attempt to postpone inevitable (eg, many promises, often to God, are made).

Depression
Reaction to many losses, emotional preparation for separation (eg, silence, withdrawn, sad, somber mood, increased contemplation, powerless, guilt, change in appetite and/or sleep patterns are common traits).

Acceptance
Coming to terms with losses and death, struggling ends, peace ensues (eg, may be less involved with others and may begin planning rest of life).

then return to deal with grief when they develop their first opportunistic infection.

Another factor that contributes to the path of the grief process is the individual's stage of psychological development. It is important to remember that an individual's chronological age is not necessarily indicative of the current psychological developmental stage. Familiarity with Erik Erikson's stages of development[13] will be helpful when working with this population. When faced with what could be a terminal and chronic disease, it is difficult for an individual who is struggling with "identity versus role diffusion" to suddenly face possible death—the final stage of development. Individuals dealing with issues of adolescence are focused in the present and struggling with the question, "Who am I?" Although they have an adult view of death, it is viewed as a reality in the very distant future. When faced with possibility of their own death, the developmental view contributes to a strong sense of anger—feeling cheated of a full, rich life when they are just on the threshold of living. Even those in the young adult stage, who have crossed the threshold and are struggling with developing careers, relationships, and families, view death in the distant future. Their rage and anger can be understood when viewed from the patient's perspective. Often these patients are just beginning to see the fruit born of hard work; they have seen others die—even members of their own families, including their children.[11,12]

Social Support

Patients often report that they are the ones to whom others turn for support and that one of the challenges of living with HIV is learning to ask for and to receive help from others. Throughout the nurse/patient relationship it is important for the nurse to help the patient identify those people whom they see as available and supportive.

Because of the chronic nature of HIV infection, the composition of the patient's support system will probably change over time. A supportive spouse, lover, or parent might become ill and lack the energy to provide the physical or emotional support needed by the patient. On the other hand, reconciliation with estranged family members or affiliation with a supportive church can increase the patient's potential for support. Various communities have established agencies to provide emotional support through buddy systems and self-help groups as well as to provide practical services such as financial assistance, transportation, and home care for people living with HIV.

References

1. Meehan J. Long-term care serves more than just elders. *Am Nurse.* 1993;25(1):10.
2. Berger KJ, Williams MB. *Fundamentals of Nursing: Collaborating for Optimal Health.* Norwalk, CT: Appleton & Lange; 1992:373–382.
3. Bradley JC, Edinburgh MA. *Communication in the Nursing Context.* 3rd ed. Norwalk, CT: Appleton & Lange; 1990:95–108.
4. Hymovich DP, Hagopian GA. *Chronic Illness in Children and Adults: A Psychosocial Approach.* Philadelphia: WB Saunders; 1992:137–169.
5. Longo DC. Communication and human behavior. In: Longo DC, Williams RA, eds. *Clinical Practice in Psychosocial Nursing Assessment and Intervention.* 2nd ed. Norwalk, CT: Appleton-Century-Crofts; 1986:1–125.
6. Thompson EA. Anxiety: a mental health vital sign. In: Longo DC, Williams RA, eds. *Clinical Practice in Psychosocial Nursing Assessment and Intervention.* 2nd ed. Norwalk, CT: Appleton-Century-Crofts; 1986:47–73.

7. Burgess AW. *Psychiatric Nursing in the Hospital and the Community.* 5th ed. Norwalk, CT: Appleton & Lange; 1990:932–935.

8. Fortinash KM, Holoday-Worret PA. *Psychiatric Nursing Plans.* St. Louis: Mosby Year Book; 1991:1–9, 257–260, 264–274.

9. Kübler-Ross E. *On Death and Dying.* New York: Macmillan; 1969:1–260.

10. Mauksch HO. The organizational context of dying. In: Kübler–Ross E. *Death: The Final Stage of Growth.* Englewood Cliffs, NJ: Prentice–Hall; 1975:7–24.

11. Leming MR, Dickinson GE. *Understanding Dying, Death, and Bereavement.* New York: Holt, Rinehart & Winston; 1985:105–137.

12. Rando TA. *Grief, Dying, and Death: Clinical Interventions for Caregivers.* Champaign, IL: Research Press Co; 1984:227–266.

13. Erikson EH. *Identity: Youth and Crisis.* New York: WW Norton & Co; 1968:104–135.

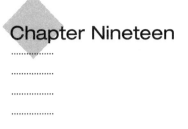

Chapter Nineteen

Outpatient Nursing

Bernadette M. Montgomerie, RN

The impact of AIDS and HIV disease on the outpatient care setting has been overwhelming and may raise some concern about the adequacy of attention to patient education and risk management. With such a large percentage of patients leaving the hospital setting with vascular access devices and complicated intravenous medication regimens for viral and fungal infections, it is important that the nurse be knowledgeable in all areas of teaching the necessary procedures and that documentation be provided to patients regarding their role expectations and "troubleshooting" guidelines (Boxes 19–1, 19–2, 19–3).

Increasingly patients are being discharged from the hospital setting early in their recovery period. Their home care, which ideally should be managed by a registered nurse, more likely becomes the responsibility of the patient, family, or friends.

■ Outpatient Procedures

Procedures that may be conducted in the outpatient setting that require nursing intervention include indwelling

■ **Box 19–1**
Patient Instructions for Drug
Administration via the Hohn Catheter

Date _____

Name _____

Medication Regimen:

　Ganciclovir (DHPG) _____ mg in 0.9%
　　sodium 100 ml _____ daily, 7 days per week

　OR

　Amphotericin B _____ mg in dextrose in
　water _____ ml daily, 7 days per week

Procedure:

Always wipe rubber stoppers with alcohol before
inserting needles or cannulas

1. Assemble materials, prepare yourself and prepare the working surface as instructed.
2. Place ganciclovir/amphotericin B bag on tubing
   and prime tubing to clear tube of air. Place blue
   threaded lock cannula on end of tube.
3. Clean catheter with alcohol. Connect needleless
   cannula to syringe and flush catheter with 10 ml
   of 0.9% sodium chloride.
4. Connect medication bag and tubing to catheter.

GANCICLOVIR: Infuse over a 1-hour period
(16 drops per minute, 8 drops per 30 seconds, or
4 drops per 15 seconds).

AMPHOTERICIN B:
4-hour infusion—Count 5 drops per 15 seconds.
3-hour infusion—Count 7 drops per 15 seconds.
2-hour infusion—Count 10 drops per 15 seconds.

———— *continued* ————

■ **Box 19–1** *(continued)*

5. When medication infusion is complete, disconnect the tubing from the catheter.

6. Clean catheter cap (rubber stopper) with alcohol. Flush catheter with 10 ml 0.9% sodium chloride.

7. Clean catheter cap with alcohol. Flush catheter with _____ ml Hep-lock solution, 100 units per ml.

8. Discard used syringes and cannulas in sharps container. Place tubing and bags in sealed plastic garbage bag.

9. Store reconstituted ganciclovir in refrigerator prior to use. Ganciclovir is stable for 14 days when stored in refrigerator. Store reconstituted amphotericin B bags in brown paper sack in refrigerator prior to use. It is stable for 14 days.

10. Inspect medication for cloudiness or floating particles before use. Notify clinician and discard if this occurs.

11. Gloves, gowns, and masks are recommended to be used by the person administering the medication.

12. Store all prefilled syringes in refrigerator prior to use.

■ Box 19-2
Patient Instructions on How to Flush (or Rinse) Catheter

It is possible that your catheter tubing could get clogged with a blood clot. To keep this from happening, you will flush your tube with a liquid called heparin. You will be provided with syringes that have been prefilled with the appropriate amount of heparin, and you will need to flush your catheter daily, after each catheter use, and each time the cap is changed.

Supplies you will need:
1. Alcohol wipes.
2. Prefilled syringe with heparin flush solution (Hep-lock).*
3. "Interlink" needleless cannula.
4. Sharps container.

Procedure:
1. Assemble supplies as above.
2. Wash and dry hands thoroughly. Use soap and water.
3. Remove the cannula from its package and attach it to the syringe without touching the exposed area. Remove any air from the syringe by gently tapping any bubbles to the top, then carefully pushing up on the barrel of the syringe until you see a droplet of liquid on the end of the cannula. Unclamp the catheter.
4. Clean the rubber stopper at the end of the catheter with an alcohol wipe.
5. Insert the cannula into the center of the rubber stopper (injection cap) and administer the heparin gently. If no resistance is felt, inject all of the

continued

■ **Box 19–2** *(continued)*

solution slowly. If resistance is felt, DO NOT FORCE—CONTACT YOUR CLINICIAN AS SOON AS POSSIBLE. Reclamp the catheter.
6. Dispose of used syringe and cannula in sharps container.

---

* *These instructions should also be followed when flushing with sodium chloride solution before and after medication infusions.*

■ **Box 19–3**
Patient Instructions on How to Change Injection Cap

The injection cap (rubber stopper) needs to be changed every 2 weeks. Wash your hands thoroughly before beginning the procedure.

1. Close the slide clamp on your catheter.
2. Peel open the package containing the new injection cap.
3. Hold the catheter in one hand near the cap. With the other hand, twist the cap by turning counterclockwise. Do not remove the rubber stopper from the plastic body.
4. Remove the plastic cover on the bottom of the new cap.
5. Twist the new cap onto the catheter tube.
6. Inject heparin solution as instructed.
7. RECLAMP THE CATHETER.

vascular access catheter care, blood transfusions, lumbar punctures, and bone marrow aspiration and biopsies. Primary responsibilities of the nurse should include patient comfort, patient education, and appropriate barrier precautions for the health care worker performing the procedure.

■ Indwelling Vascular Access Catheters

The principal life-threatening complication in any patient who has a vascular catheter is septicemia. In a patient with AIDS, the risk is multiplied many times. Because of repeated infections that result in the need for a future hospitalization to remove the infected Groshong, Hickman, or Port-a-Cath catheter and replace it in the operating room, clinicians have searched for other options. One of these is the Hohn central venous catheter (Figs. 19–1, 19–2). This catheter is introduced percutaneously, and the procedure can be performed at the patient's bedside under local anesthesia. The catheter was designed for short-term use and as a rule should be replaced after 2 or 3 months. Since this is not a "tunneled" catheter, it can easily be removed in the outpatient setting by a trained registered nurse.

Some clinicians who use the Hohn catheter have concluded that dressing changes can be performed less frequently than the usual every 72 hours. With this catheter, patients are required to return to the clinic setting to have a dressing change performed once weekly (Box 19–4). Therefore, patients do not need to worry about doing their own dressing care, and strict controls can be followed regarding the specific care to minimize contamination. In our clinical experience, it has been found that the rate of infection has decreased considerably since we adopted this method of care.

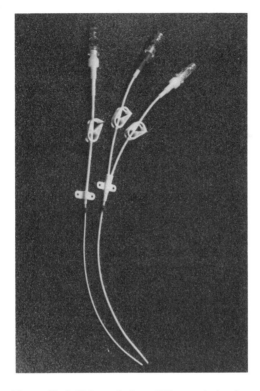

Figure 19–1. Hohn catheters. With permission from Bard Access Systems.

Since Hohn catheters do not have a valve at their proximal end, daily flushing with heparin is necessary. Patients are taught to flush the catheter with 200 units of Hep-lock (100 units per cc) solution using prefilled syringes and attaching "Interlink cannulas," which are plastic tips that pierce the "Interlink injection cap" without the use of a needle. This has been found to be a helpful safety standard, particularly when dealing with

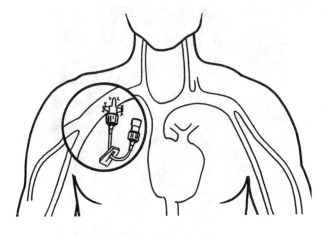

Figure 19–2. Placement of Hohn catheter.

patients who have CMV retinitis and compromised visual acuity. The catheter is also flushed with 10 cc of sodium chloride before and after administration of any intravenous medications using the same "Interlink" system.

■ Blood Transfusion

Standing orders are often utilized for blood transfusion procedures (Box 19–5). Despite increasingly accurate cross-matching precautions, transfusion reactions can, and often do, occur. Circulatory overload and hemolytic, allergic, febrile, and pyrogenic reactions can occur in any patient receiving a blood transfusion. In the HIV/AIDS population, who often require frequent transfusion of blood products, intravenous Lasix (furosemide) is often administered after each unit of blood to lessen the possi-

■ Box 19–4

Patient Instructions for
Changing Dressing

The type of dressing used should only need to be changed on a weekly basis. However, if the dressing should become soiled or is just coming off the skin, it should be changed more frequently. Before leaving the hospital, you will be supplied with several dressing kits.

Catheter Care kit containing the following supplies:

1. Surgeons masks (2)
2. Surgeons gloves (1 pair)
3. Gauze 4 × 4s (10)
4. Package swabsticks, alcohol (3 sticks)
5. Package swabsticks, povidone-iodine (3 sticks)
6. Package ointment, povidone-iodine
7. Gauze 2 × 2s (2)
8. Gauze 2 × 2, split (1)
9. Povidone-iodine pad (1)
10. Interlink injection cap (1)
11. Dry swab sticks (3)
12. Skin prep pad (1)
13. Op-site (transparent) dressing 10 × 14 (1)
    Also: Micropore tape

Procedure:

1. Gather all supplies.
2. Wash and dry hands thoroughly. Use soap and water.
3. Open Catheter Care kit by touching only the outside of the wrapper. Place on top of a clean dry sheet or towel.

—— *continued* ——

■ **Box 19-4** *(continued)*

4. Remove masks carefully. Use one for patient, the other for the caregiver.
5. Remove old dressing and discard in appropriate manner.
6. Wash hands again.
7. Inspect catheter site carefully. If any redness, swelling or drainage is noted, or if a suture has become loose, notify your clinician as soon as possible.
8. Carefully remove sterile gloves and put on by:
   a) Grabbing the turned back cuff of one of the gloves. Pull the glove on your free hand. Be careful not to touch the outside of the glove below the cuff.
   b) Using the gloved hand, slide the fingers of that hand under the folded cuff of the next glove and pull it on to your hand.
   c) You can now use either hand to gently arrange your fingers in the gloves. DO NOT TOUCH ANYTHING before you go on to the next steps. (Holding your hands above the level of your waist will help you to remember this.)
9. Open the sterile field containing the rest of the items.
10. Use your nondominant hand to hold the end of the catheter. Your other hand will do most of the work. Use one of the sterile 4 × 4s to prevent contamination of your sterile glove.
    First, take one of the alcohol swabsticks and clean around the catheter exit site working outward in a widening circle. Repeat this two more times using a new swabstick each time.

continued

■ **Box 19–4** *(continued)*

Repeat this procedure using the brown iodine swabsticks.

Next, using the brown iodine wipe, clean the tubing from the exit site toward the injection cap. Using one or more of the sterile 4 × 4s, pat the entire area dry.

11. Take a dry swabstick and apply some of the antiseptic ointment over the insertion and suture sites, using a different swabstick for each site.
12. Take the skin prep pad and wipe the skin around the catheter site, but not immediately surrounding it.
13. Take the 2 × 2 split gauze and place under the catheter hub.
14. Cover this with the other 2 × 2s provided.
15. Apply transparent dressing over this.
16. Secure excess catheter and injection cap to chest with tape.

Person to contact for questions or problems:

■ Box 19-5
Standing Orders for Blood Transfusions

Please check or fill in appropriate response.

1. Allergies: _____

2. Type & cross for _____ units PRBCs
   or
   Type & cross done _____ (date)

3. Pt. to receive transfusion within 24 hours
   _____ Yes _____ No
   may schedule transfusion as convenient
   _____ Yes _____ No

4. Transfuse each unit over 1.5 to 2.0 hours

5. Prior to transfusion premedicate with:
   Tylenol 650 mg p.o.
   Benadryl 50 mg p.o.

6. Give Lasix 10 mg SIVP after each unit
   _____ Yes _____ No
   Hold Lasix if BP below _____ or pulse
   above _____

7. May repeat Tylenol 650 mg q 3–4 hours prn for
   temp greater than 101°F.

8. Please obtain CBC posttransfusion
   _____ Yes _____ No

9. For problems, call Dr._____
   Beeper #_____   Phone #_____

bility of circulatory overload. As with any patient receiving transfusions, the nurse must exercise care in frequent monitoring of vital signs as well as fluid intake and output patterns. Documentation of this as well as any transfusion reaction and treatment should be done.

■ Lumbar Puncture/Bone Marrow Aspiration and Biopsy

The outpatient clinic nurse is often required to assist with these procedures, which require sterile technique and careful patient positioning. The nurse should first ensure that the patient understands the procedure to ease anxiety and to ensure cooperation. A consent form must be signed indicating that the patient has received adequate explanation of the procedure and its possible advantages and disadvantages. The nurse should check the patient's history for hypersensitivity to the local anesthetic and provide a sedative, as ordered, before the procedure.

Both the health care worker performing the procedure as well as the assistant must wear appropriate protective barrier gown, mask, goggles, and sterile gloves. Care should be exercised when handling the instruments and body fluids obtained from the patient. During the procedure, the nurse should be aware of any signs of adverse reaction: elevated pulse rate, pallor, or clammy skin. Bleeding and infection are potentially life-threatening complications that may result from either of these procedures. The nurse should immediately alert the clinician performing the procedure to any significant changes in the patient's condition.

Finally, the nurse is responsible for charting the time, date, location, and patient's tolerance of the procedure and any specimens obtained.

■ Patient Education

Patients with AIDS and HIV disease present nursing with innumerable challenges and involve all areas of functioning: physical, psychological, economic, and spiritual. Also, because this is a highly publicized disease, patient advocacy is essential to protect patients from unwarranted intrusion into their privacy.

Because this disease most often impacts early in life and is known to be terminal, many patients develop a loss of hope early in the disease process. This loss of hope puts enormous responsibilities on nurses to ensure that the care and support they give is of the highest standards and offers the best possible quality of life.

Much of the fear experienced by patients results from their not knowing what is being done to them. Simple explanations of procedures and nursing care will alleviate this and help involve the patient in his or her own care and so gain their cooperation.

Chapter Twenty

....
....
....
....

PREVENTION

BARBARA ANN LYONS, MA, PA-C
PEGGY VALENTINE, EdD, PA-C

At present, there is no known cure for AIDS, no vaccine available for prevention, and no proven method for eliminating the infectivity of the HIV carrier. For these reasons, great emphasis must be placed on preventing the transmission of HIV.

■ Modes of Transmission

The major modes of transmission for HIV are sexual contact with an infected person and contact with contaminated blood, predominately through the sharing of needles and syringes by injecting drug users. There is no evidence of transmission through casual contact (eg, food, dishes, toilets, or sneezing). Although HIV has been isolated from body fluids and tissues including blood, semen, saliva, tears, breast milk, urine, lymph nodes, brain tissue, cerebrospinal fluid, and bone marrow, only blood and semen harbor moderate to high concentrations of virus and hence are the only body fluids to date that have been epidemiologically linked to transmission.

Since many unknowns still exist regarding HIV infection, it seems prudent to consider all body fluids, tissues, secretions, and excretions from all patients as potentially infectious, particularly if they contain blood. Parenteral or mucous membrane contact with these substances should be avoided. Current universal blood and body fluid precautions state that all body fluids from all patients are to be treated as if infective.

■ Reducing Risk of HIV Transmission

Guidelines have been developed by the Centers for Disease Control and Prevention (CDC) and the Occupational Safety and Health Administration (OSHA) to minimize the risk of exposure to blood and body fluids. The following of these guidelines should greatly reduce the transmission of HIV and HBV to individuals and health care workers (HCWs).

Individual Risk Reduction

For the individual, many methods are recommended to reduce the risk of HIV transmission. Overall, education and gaining correct knowledge concerning the pathophysiology of HIV and its transmission are of the utmost importance since individuals need to know the facts about the disease and the behaviors that help prevent its spread. Most individuals at risk for HIV infection participate in at least one of several risky behaviors: anal intercourse, sex with multiple partners, injecting drug use (IDU), medical treatment with blood or blood products, or sex with a person who participates in any of the first four mentioned behaviors. Infants are at risk for transmission from their HIV-infected mother while in utero, at delivery, and postpartum.

Sexual contact among homosexuals has been the leading risk factor for acquiring HIV. Risky sex acts include unprotected receptive anal intercourse and oral sex. These types of sex acts may cause local tissue injury, which would be a portal of entry for the virus from the partner's semen. Some homosexuals have multiple sex partners, thereby giving them additional risk. For patients who are homosexual, discussion of their sexual practices is essential. Upon evaluation of the specific practices, protective measures should be discussed. For example, a patient participating in receptive anal intercourse may choose to abstain from the activity. Alternatively, condoms may be used.

Having multiple sexual partners, heterosexual and/or homosexual, is also considered a risky behavior. As the number of people involved increases, so does the risk of one or more of them carrying HIV. Although some people may have had sex with a few different partners, others may have had sex with hundreds of different people. Prostitutes may not want to inform their clients about their health, and instances of unprotected sex may occur. Prevention of the risk from multiple partners includes patient awareness of the risk involved. The patient may decrease the number of future partners or may choose to use condoms to prevent the spread of the virus.

For injecting drug users, the risk is from blood contact through sharing and/or reuse of hypodermic needles and syringes. IDU is defined as any route in which the skin is broken with a needle and includes intravenous, intraarterial, intramuscular, and subdermal routes of injection. Patients who participate in IDU may benefit from a number of preventive measures. Drug rehabilitation is possible for some patients who are motivated to stop their drug use. For patients who cannot or will not cease IDU, safety measures that may help decrease the spread of HIV include not sharing needles, cleaning used syringes and needles with bleach solution, or needle exchange programs. Some patients will engage in prostitution to procure drugs and will be at higher risk than from IDU alone.

Even if they do not participate in any risky behaviors themselves, some people may be at risk for acquiring HIV if their sexual partners engage in any risky behaviors. Prevention of HIV in these individuals would include the knowledge of the risks of their sexual partners. For all people with a current or past history of homosexual sexual activity, multiple sexual partners, IDU, and/or blood or blood product treatment, the employment of "safer sex" techniques with their sexual partners may help prevent the spread of HIV. Sexual abstinence is the only completely safe method to prevent the sexual transmission of HIV. Since this choice is not popular, prevention methods termed "safer sex" techniques have been outlined. Although the use of "safer sex" techniques will not prevent the transmission of HIV completely, they do afford some level of protection. A noninclusive list of "safer sex" techniques includes abstaining from risky sex acts, including anal or vaginal intercourse; the use of a latex condom during risky sex acts; use of the spermicide nonoxinol-9; and the use of massage and touching.

Patients who have been treated with blood or blood product transfusion may be at a higher risk for HIV. Prior to late 1985, the general blood supply was not adequately tested for the presence of HIV antibodies. Additionally, blood clotting factors given to hemophiliacs were also not tested for the presence of HIV. Consequently, many patients requiring blood transfusions or clotting factor administration were inadvertently given HIV. Since blood donors are now screened prior to donation for any risk factors for HIV and the blood supply is tested for HIV antibodies, the risk of transmission of HIV is much lower and was estimated to be between 1 per 40,000 and 1 per

150,000 units infused in 1989.[1] Patients who received blood transfusions or blood clotting factors prior to 1985, pending the knowledge of their HIV status, may abstain from sexual contact or employ "safer sex" techniques. Since there remains a risk of HIV transmission from blood transfusion, patients currently receiving blood transfusions may choose the same options. For patients who will need blood transfusion or clotting factors in the future, prevention methods include a number of options such as preoperative autologous blood donation, hemodilution, perioperative blood salvage, and the use of recombinant coagulation factors, recombinant hematopoietic growth factors, and red cell substitutes.[1]

Transmission of HIV to the fetus and newborn is possible. For the known HIV-positive woman, prevention methods may include using contraception to prevent pregnancy and abstaining from breast feeding. Any woman of childbearing age who is sexually active should understand the risk of transmission of HIV to her future children and may want to practice "safer sex" techniques to keep from becoming infected. More details on the prevention of the transmission of HIV from mother to child are found in Chapter 13.

Health Care Worker Risk Reduction

For the health care worker, OSHA guidelines[2] include the use of personal protective equipment (PPE) to decrease the risk from blood or other potentially infectious materials. Gloves, gowns, laboratory coats, face shields or masks, and eye protection are included in PPE. The choice of what PPE is appropriate for each HCW job activity needs to be defined. If a HCW is performing a job task where hand contact with blood or other infectious material is expected, gloves must be worn. For most HCW tasks, single-use gloves are appropriate. These latex gloves are disposed of after one use. If the HCW is allergic to latex, hypoallergic gloves must be provided. Gloving is required for almost all phlebotomy situations. The only exception to the rule is in voluntary blood donation centers, where gloving for phlebotomy is not required. A HCW in a voluntary blood center may choose to use gloves at any time; however, they must use gloves if they have cuts, scratches, or breaks in their skin, while training, or when it is believed that contamination may occur.

For clinical activities where splashes, sprays, splatters, or droplets of potentially infectious material pose a hazard through the eyes, nose, or mouth, face protection should be used. These protection methods include the use of goggles and masks, glasses with solid side shields and masks, or chin-length face shields. These measures would be appropriate for activities including, for example, the use of jet lavage for wound cleansing and tub therapy for debridement of burn wounds. For clinical situations where gross contamination is expected, more extensive coverings such as gowns, aprons, surgical caps/hoods, and shoe covers or boots are needed in addition to gloves and face protection. This level of protection would be needed for clinical activities such as orthopedic surgery or autopsy.

After removal of any PPE, hands must be washed with soap and water as soon as feasible. If access to soap and water is delayed, interim hand-cleansing measures such as use of moist towelettes may be employed followed by timely appropriate hand washing. Used protective clothing and equipment must be placed in designated containers for storage, decontamination, or disposal.

HCWs with weeping dermatitis or exudative lesions should refrain from all patient contact until the condition resolves. Even though saliva has not been implicated as a source of HIV transmission, limiting the use of mouth-to-mouth resuscitation seems wise. Where emergency resuscitation is predictable, mouthpieces, resuscitation bags

(Ambu bags), or other ventilation assist devises should be available. In the event of a skin or mucous membrane contact with a potentially infectious body fluid, the body area of contact is to be washed with soap and water. In the event of eye contact, copious irrigation with water is recommended. When HCWs experience parenteral exposures, needle sticks, scalpel cuts, or mucous membrane exposure, testing for HIV and hepatitis should be performed (see Chapter 5).

Depending on their specific job requirements, HCWs may be responsible for decontamination of work surface areas or equipment that may involve exposure to blood. Work areas are to be cleaned when (1) surfaces are obviously contaminated; (2) after any spill of blood or other potentially infective body fluid; and (3) at any time the worker leaves a potentially contaminated area, including breaks, meals, or at a shift's end. Each employer is responsible for developing guidelines for decontamination that specify the methods of decontamination used for different surfaces, types of contamination present, and types of procedures done in the area. In addition to commercially available germicides, household bleach (sodium hypochlorite) in a dilution of 1:100 or 1:10 is an effective method depending on the amount of organic material present. Some medical devices may corrode from continual exposure to the 1:10 bleach solution so that commercial germicides may need to be used. OSHA also recommends that HCWs refrain from eating, drinking, smoking, applying lipstick or lip balm, and handling contact lenses in areas where blood or body fluid exposure is possible.

Prompt disposal of all medical sharps, including needles and scalpels, will minimize stick and cut exposures in HCWs. Containers for disposable and reusable sharps that are puncture resistant and leakproof should be located close by the area where sharps are used. The location of the containers should eliminate the need to set the needle or scalpel on a surface after its use or the sticking of contaminated needles into a mattress of a patient bed or gurney prior to proper disposal. In most clinical situations, recapping, bending, or removal of needles *should not* be performed. These techniques account for the majority of needle sticks and cuts. For testing that requires the needle to be left in place, such as arterial blood gas determination, recapping, bending, or removal of the needle should be performed by a mechanical device or by using the one-hand recapping technique. The use of both hands to recap a needle is to be avoided. The one-hand technique involves use of the needle itself to slip into the needle cap. Pressure on a hard surface may complete the closure. Alternatively, tongs or forceps could be used to place the cap on the needle. Even when performed using an approved method, recapping of needles is limited to those situations when recapping is required.

HCWs are forbidden to handle potentially contaminated broken glass by hand, even if gloves are worn. Glass fragments are to be collected using a brush and dustpan, tongs, or forceps and disposed of in a contaminated sharps container.

Laundry that is contaminated with blood or other potentially infective material should be handled as little as possible and with a minimum of agitation. All soiled linen should be bagged in the area of use and transported to the laundry facility. No sorting or prewashing should be done in patient care areas.

Despite adherence to the principles of universal precautions, certain invasive surgical and dental procedures (ie, cardiothoracic, obstetric/gynecological, and oral procedures) have been implicated in the transmission of HBV from infected HCWs to patients and should thus be considered as posing a high risk of exposure.[3] Exposure-prone procedures may also be implicated in the transmission of HIV. Characteristics of such procedures include digital palpation of a needle tip in a body cavity or the simultaneous presence of the HCW's fingers and a needle or other sharp instrument or object in a poorly visualized or highly confined anatomic site.[3] To minimize the risk of HIV or HBV transmission, the CDC recommends the following measures[3]:

- All HCWs should adhere to the universal precautions already mentioned.
- Currently available data provide no basis for recommendations to restrict the practice of HCWs infected with HIV or HBV who perform invasive procedures not identified as posing a high risk of exposure, provided that the infected HCWs practice recommended surgical or dental technique and comply with universal precautions and current recommendations for sterilization/disinfection.
- Exposure-prone procedures should be identified by the medical/surgical/dental organizations and institutions at which the procedures are performed.
- HCWs who perform exposure-prone procedures should know their HIV antibody status. HCWs who perform exposure-prone procedures and who do not have serologic evidence of immunity to HBV from vaccination or from previous infection should know their HBsAg status and, if that is positive, should also know their HBeAg status.
- HCWs who are infected with HIV or HBV (and are HBeAg positive) should not perform high-risk procedures unless they have sought counsel from an expert review panel and been advised under what circumstances, if any, they may continue to perform these procedures. Such circumstances would include notifying prospective patients of the HCW's seropositivity before they undergo exposure-prone invasive procedures.

- Mandatory testing of HCWs for HIV antibody, HBsAg, or HBeAg is not recommended. The current assessment of the risk that infected HCWs will transmit HIV or HBV to patients during exposure-prone procedures does not support the diversion of resources that would be required to implement mandatory testing programs. Compliance by HCWs with recommendations can be increased through education, training, and appropriate confidentiality safeguards.

The guidelines for HCWs are frequently updated, and it should be noted that clinicians will need to keep informed of any future changes.

■ Prevention in Minority Populations

Because the three largest ethnic minority groups—African- Americans, Hispanics, and Asian-Americans—represent over 30% of the U.S. population and, when combined, represent over 46% of reported AIDS cases,[4] a separate discussion regarding prevention in these populations is warranted. In addition, there is an overrepresentation of women, children, and heterosexuals with AIDS from these ethnic minority groups. Over 73% of women and 78% of children and heterosexuals with AIDS are African-American or Hispanic.[4] The HIV seroprevalence rate for Asian-Americans, Native Americans, and Pacific Islanders has been relatively low; they continue to be underrepresented in proportion to their total numbers in the U.S. population. However, from 1989 to 1990 the number of Native American AIDS cases increased faster than that for any other racial or ethnic group. It is thought that these groups are still in the early stages of a growing HIV epidemic.[5]

A history of IDU tends to be the major risk factor for the disparity noted in African-American and Hispanic populations. Although drug use is prevalent among all race groups, IDU is more highly associated with HIV seroprevalence among these groups. This high-risk behavior, which may or may not be known to a sexual partner, increases the chance of heterosexual and, subsequently, neonatal transmission.[5]

Despite targeted HIV prevention programs, the number of AIDS cases in minority groups continues to escalate. Some members of these groups do not believe the prevention messages and continue to engage in high-risk behavior; others may have more immediate needs of daily survival. Before designing and implementing HIV prevention strategies for minority groups, the provider should consider certain sociocultural issues.

Theories of the Epidemiology of HIV

In some minority communities, there are those who believe that HIV was purposely introduced into the community by the government to control population growth. It is believed that the virus was created through genetic engineering to "kill off" undesirable gays and minorities. The theory that "AIDS originated in Africa" may be interpreted to mean that HIV came from persons of African descent, and thus that they are to be blamed for the disease.[5] Condom promotion is seen by some as population control imposed by the majority so as to decrease the minority population. Others view needle exchange programs as a way to promote drug use in the African-American community. These beliefs and perceptions create barriers for HIV prevention programs in that those who believe these theories may not heed government prevention messages.[5–7]

When designing and implementing an HIV prevention program in the African-American community, the clinician should first discern what beliefs and perceptions are held. Patients should be encouraged to discuss their feelings and concerns about these issues. Sometimes sharing a story with a philosophical meaning may generate discussion. One story sometimes shared is that of the snake in the house. Should we expend our energy on asking where it came from or should we rather focus our efforts on getting it out of the house? The provider can also show concern and assist the patient in identifying ways to lower the risk of HIV and other sexually transmitted diseases.

Fear of Homosexuality/Bisexuality

Despite the gay awareness movement of the past two decades, many ethnic minorities do not support the concept of homosexuality and look down on those who are openly gay. Therefore, some minority males choose to remain "closeted" or to engage in bisexual relationships. This lifestyle may be burdensome enough, and the male who is a member of a minority, gay, and afflicted with AIDS may well feel overburdened. Unfortunately, there are few support services in minority communities for gay persons infected with HIV. It is common for African-American males to misrepresent their mode of HIV exposure to avoid stigma and maintain support from family and friends.[5,7] The provider may assist the patient through referral to national AIDS minority organizations (see Chapter 16). Some of these organizations provide educational services to the gay community and can provide information on local support groups.

Another issue of importance to the provider is how members of minority groups define homosexuality. For example, Hispanic men may define a homosexual male as the receptive partner in anal intercourse, and the insertive partner may not be considered homosexual.[5] In establishing a common language, it is recommended that providers ask the patient if he has sex with men, with women, or with both.[8]

Bisexuality is an important risk factor to be considered in the Hispanic community, and women partners of bisexual males may be at increased risk for acquiring HIV. In some cases, Hispanic women perceive their relationships as characterized by a power imbalance and thus consider themselves limited in their ability to reduce this risk.[5] In working with women who feel unempowered in their relationships, the provider can recommend various support groups that build self-esteem. The provider can also identify resource persons from federal, state, and local governments and community-based organizations to work with the patient.

Disbelief of Prevention Messages

Minority communities have had negative experiences with public health groups in the past, which may cause mistrust of HIV prevention messages today. For example, many remember the Tuskegee Syphilis Study in which some African-American males with syphilis were allowed to progress to an advanced stage of the disease without adequate treatment.[9] This example and others have caused minorities to become mistrustful and to experience a certain amount of discomfort when discussing the impact of HIV/AIDS on their communities. Since the Tuskegee Study, improvements have certainly been made in the research environment to protect human subjects. However, beliefs and perceptions are slow to change—indeed, certain events, however appalling, must remain in our consciousness so that the same mistakes will not be repeated.

The building of trust in patient–provider relationships comes about through a series of interactions and through open and honest communication. One should not always assume that minority providers are best able to relate to minority patients with HIV seropositivity. Minority patients may in fact not be more trusting of minority providers of the same culture; some fear that minority providers are more likely to pass judgment upon them. In any case, it is important to convince the patient that he or she has the provider's support and trust. Sometimes sharing personal information equalizes the balance of power and can help to build a more trusting relationship. This sharing should ideally take place during the first patient–provider interaction.[5]

Poverty

Minorities are disproportionately represented at income levels associated with poverty. They have higher rates of unemployment and lower incomes than white Americans. Most African-Americans and Hispanics at risk for HIV are of lower socioeconomic status. These minorities are less likely to seek early treatment for AIDS, tend to seek access to the health care system later in the course of HIV-related illnesses, and die sooner from AIDS than do whites.[5]

Clearly the provider cannot erase poverty and improve access to health care for all; however, he or she can nevertheless exert a positive impact on minority communities by working with their members to promote healthier lifestyles. Minorities often do not know what resources are available outside the community, especially if they do not speak English. The provider can point individuals to local resources that provide free or reduced-fee services. Community forums that involve social service agencies can be arranged to disseminate information on health care services to the public.

Differences in Language and Culture and Their Effect on Communication

In some instances, HIV prevention literature is not communicated effectively to minority populations. HIV prevention programs are further hampered in minority groups because of the presence of diverse communities with culturally specific attitudes and beliefs, including those pertaining to the roles of males and females. For example, in disseminating HIV prevention messages in Native American communities, it is important that the messages be delivered by members of the communities.[5] Similarly, Pacific islanders may not believe or trust messages delivered by individuals from outside their communities. It may therefore be more effective to train outreach workers in these communities to provide HIV education.[5]

Language is a barrier for certain minority groups in gaining access to HIV education because of the variety of languages and dialects among those groups. This is a particular problem in the Asian-American/Pacific islander group and among Hispanic groups. In addition, health care providers may be unable to translate or provide appropriately translated materials. Whenever possible, materials should be written at the appropriate grade level and depict the language, culture, and style of communication of the targeted group.[5,6]

It is also suggested that HIV information specific to women be disseminated. Since minority women face issues involving their cultural roles as spouses and mothers differently from men, separate programs may be needed.

In conclusion, when implementing or participating in HIV prevention programs for minorities, the provider should gain an appreciation of the patient's life experiences, values, and belief systems. This may require a series of visits in the clinical setting and preferably in the domestic environment. Through learning about the individual patient, the provider will have a better understanding of how to disseminate HIV prevention information. Providers should consider the social, cultural, and economic factors that influence HIV prevention in minorities. Providers should also be aware of their own limitations, strengths, and weaknesses and should utilize all available resources, including local health departments and grantees of the CDC and National Institutes of Health AIDS Education Training Centers.

References

1. OSHA Instruction CPC 2-2-44C, Enforcement procedures for the occupational exposure to bloodborne pathogens standard, 29 CFR 1910.1030, March 6, 1992.

2. Healthy People 2000, DHHS, PHS, Superintendent of Documents, U.S. Government Printing Office, 1990.

3. Centers for Disease Control. Recommendations for preventing transmission of human immunodeficiency virus and hepatitis B virus to patients during exposure-prone invasive procedures. *MMWR.* 1991; 40(RR-8):1–9.

4. Centers for Disease Control. *HIV/AIDS Surveillance Report.* February 1993:1–23.

5. National Commission on AIDS. *The Challenge of HIV/AIDS in Communities of Color.* Washington, DC: 1992.

6. Peterson JL, Marin G. Issues in the prevention of AIDS among black and hispanic men. *Am Psychol.* 1988;43:871–877.

7. Dalton HL. Living with AIDS: part II. *Daedalus.* 1989;118:205–227.

8. Mann J, Tarantola DJM, Netter TW. *AIDS in the World.* Cambridge, MA: Harvard University Press; 1992.

9. Thomas SB, Quinn SC. The Tuskegee syphilis study, 1932 to 1972: implications for HIV education and AIDS risk education programs in the black community. *Am J Public Health.* 1991;81:1498–1503.

Chapter Twenty-One

SOCIAL AND PSYCHOLOGICAL ASPECTS OF AIDS

JOHN G. BRUHN, PhD

AIDS has had profound medical, political, and social ramifications. AIDS has become a political issue in both the public and private sectors, and serious social problems have resulted, both from the fears of contagion and from the initial appearance of the syndrome among stigmatized minorities. Homophobia has increased at a time otherwise characterized by greater acceptance of homosexuality. Significant psychological concerns have arisen among health care workers as a result of prejudice and fears of contagion. These issues have added to the psychological and social burdens of patients with AIDS, who face a debilitating disease with a poor prognosis.

■ Psychological Adaptation

The psychological adaptation to any severe life-threatening disease depends upon factors derived from three major areas. These factors are medical (symptoms, clinical course, and complications, particularly of the central nervous system); psychological (personality and coping; interpersonal support); and sociocultural (social stigma attached to the disease and affected groups). The frequent complications of the central nervous system may impair the patient's behavior. As evidence of the link between the central nervous and immune systems continues to grow, the implications for hypothesizing a relationship between stress and the clinical course of AIDS becomes more promising—as do the indications for using stress reduction strategies. There is some evidence that risk reduction measures may positively affect the clinical course.

The medical or disease-related factors are the primary determinants of adaptation because they constitute the altered physical state and medical circumstances to which the patients must adapt. These key factors in AIDS are the impact of diagnosis; common symptoms and events in the clinical course; nature of the frequent psychological distress and psychiatric disorders; central nervous system complications; and the responses of care givers.

The diagnosis of AIDS is a catastrophic event because it is known to have a rapid downhill course, no definitive treatment, and an extremely poor prognosis. The diagnosis is usually made over the course of weeks to months, as the patient fears that AIDS may be the cause of frequent infections, swollen nodes, and general malaise. After a diagnosis of AIDS is made, each new symptom, infection, loss of weight, or fatigue is regarded as a sign of potential progression of disease. The characteristic skin lesions of Kaposi's sarcoma, when present, provide visible evidence of the diagnosis. Transmission of AIDS through sexual contact or body fluids often leads to self-imposed or clinician-recommended limitation of social and intimate contacts. Guidelines for "safe sex" may require marked alteration of sexual behavior and the need to reveal one's medical status to partners. Pressure to accept a monogamous relationship or celibacy may be difficult.

The sociocultural burden of the diagnosis of AIDS results from several sources. The social stigma associated with the contagious aspect causes altered behavior in others, including avoidance of physical and social contact. Although this is painful enough for adults, even children with AIDS have become isolated from schools and from other children by frightened parents.

The diagnosis may force the patient's identification as a likely member of a stigmatized minority (homosexual, drug user, or recent immigrant). Families may abruptly learn of a lifestyle they find difficult to accept. In the largest risk group, homosexual and bisexual men, the diagnosis may create a crisis in which an otherwise private sexual preference is revealed. Drug users are already the objects of negative societal attitudes and have little advocacy in society. Haitians, even long-term residents, have been the focus of prejudicial treatment. Hemophiliacs and recipients of blood transfusions receive the most sympathetic response because of the perceived random nature of the exposure. Although some persons have acquired AIDS through blood transfusions, the main tendency of the public is "to blame the victim" for having AIDS. Sexual transmission of AIDS by prostitutes may cause an association of the disease with this socially ostracized group.

Patients with AIDS are vulnerable to rejection and feelings of guilt, arising from concerns that their behavior, particularly sexual, may endanger others. The emotions associated with harboring a contagious agent may cause the patient to feel like an outcast. Discrimination has occurred in housing, jobs, health care, and public assistance, from both fear of contagion and prejudice. Irrational fears and negative responses of the public are a continuing problem confronted daily by patients, families, and advocacy groups.

One of the most disruptive complications of AIDS is its impact on supportive relationships. Whether the family knows about and accepts a patient's homosexuality should be ascertained by the care giver. The onset of AIDS also may force disclosure of previously disguised drug use in drug-addicted patients, which may weaken family support. The stigma attached to AIDS affects all patients, including children, women, and military service personnel.

Patients in the initial crisis stage of AIDS typically have difficulty retaining information and may distort what they are told regarding their illness. Contact with support services such as crisis counseling, legal and financial assistance, and psychotherapy should begin as early as possible.

■ Psychological Distress and Psychiatric Disorders

The psychological and psychiatric sequelae of AIDS are modified by psychological factors that characterize the person's previous level of psychological adjustment and social (interpersonal) support. Presence of a personality disorder, as in intravenous drug users, or of a previous major psychiatric disorder is more apt to result in severe psychological symptoms and a maladaptive response to the stresses of illness. The availability of social support is especially crucial because of the need for both physical and social assistance. Both homosexuals and drug users may have to face illness with less support, especially from their estranged families. The drain on friends who accept their lifestyle can be great. In fact, as the illness progresses, the primary support of many patients may be the crisis support groups and other patients with HIV. Some common psychological symptoms are listed in Table 21–1.

TABLE 21–1. COMMON TYPES OF PSYCHOLOGICAL DISTRESS IN HIV-INFECTED PATIENTS

Anxiety: Uncertainty about disease, its progression and treatment; anxiety about any new symptoms; anxiety about prognosis and impending death; hyperventilation, panic attacks.

Depression: Sadness, helplessness, lowered self-esteem, guilt, worthlessness, hopelessness, suicidal thoughts, social withdrawal, expressions of "giving up"; difficulty sleeping, loss of appetite.

Feelings of isolation and reduced social support; rejection by family and others. The lack of visitors when hospitalized may confirm these feelings.

Anger at self and others; hostility toward care givers; refusal to cooperate with care givers.

Fears about who knows or will know about the illness.

Worry about finances, loss of job, living arrangements, transportation.

Embarrassment about stigma of AIDS; denial of sexual habits.

Denial of drug abuse history.

The major form of psychological distress is preoccupation with illness and with the potential for a rapidly declining course to death. The same issues raised by the diagnosis of cancer and other diseases with high rates of fatal outcomes are raised by AIDS. A normal stress response is seen at diagnosis, characterized by disbelief, numbness, and denial and followed by anger and acute turmoil with disruptive anxiety and depressive symptoms. The anxiety and uncertainty about the disease process, clinical course, possible treatment, and outcome continue. Patients are fearful when any new physical symptom develops because it may signal progression of the disease. Hypochondriacal concerns about body function also occur. Anxiety symptoms may take the form of panic attacks, agitation, insomnia, tension, anorexia, and tachycardia.

The symptoms of depression are also prominent. The patient's mood is characterized by sadness, hopelessness, and helplessness. Guilt, low self-esteem, worthlessness, and anticipatory grief are common with social withdrawal and isolation. The idea of suicide if the disease progresses is common in most patients, especially those who have seen friends die of AIDS. Anger directed toward the illness, medical care, discrimination, and public response to the disease is often intense. Expectation of rejection by others, often the result of actual experiences, produces suspiciousness of the motivation of others.

■ Response of Care Givers

A critical factor in quality of care is the attitude and responses of care givers (all persons providing direct care to patients). Several psychological issues that usually arise separately are combined in the treatment of AIDS in such a way that they create unusually difficult problems. Identification with and sense of personal vulnerability to disease and death are elicited by taking care of young healthy persons who face rapid physical deterioration and death. The fear of contagion was most frightening when the disease was first diagnosed, because guidelines that assured protection from AIDS had not yet been formulated. The large numbers of patients with AIDS in large urban hospitals can cause care givers to become overtaxed, stressed, fatigued, and fearful of being overwhelmed by the burden of the intensive complicated care. Negative social attitudes and personal prejudices, especially homophobia, can arise, as can negative attitudes toward drug users and Haitian immigrants.

Considerable information about these issues has been developed by consultation-liaison psychiatry in relation to other diseases and is applicable to AIDS as well.

An understanding of care givers' response to the care of patients with a likely fatal disease comes largely from cancer care. Hospital staff need the opportunity to discuss their feelings about "special" patients with whom identification has occurred. These feelings are usually centered around anticipatory grieving for patients who will die; actual grief with the death of patients; and anger and frustration with the negative responses of others. Care givers need instruction in how to recognize delirium and account for changes in these patient's ability to adhere to procedures and treatment.

The fear of contagion is best managed by providing up-to-date information about universal precautions. The panic among medical staff, with inappropriate behavior based on irrational fears, has diminished as institutions have promulgated Public Health Service guidelines similar to those for hepatitis B, and provided forums for clarifying misinformation from many sources. Meetings also serve to air concerns about institutional allocation of resources, organization or AIDS services, and burden to care givers.

Personal interaction with AIDS patients may elicit otherwise masked attitudes of homophobia and negative views of drug users and patients from other cultures or different lifestyles. Care givers must be encouraged to explore personal reactions, because it is important that patients feel free to discuss their lifestyle and sexual preference and practices. Ability to openly discuss sexuality is clearly a factor in the relationship between staff and patients that provides emotional support and understanding. The need to discuss sexual precautions and answer questions of lovers and family requires that the staff member feel comfortable in these discussions. The same need applies to drug users. If negative attitudes preclude appropriate interaction, the care giver should ask to be replaced by another who can openly discuss these issues.

■ Management Guidelines

The facts outlined previously suggest several guidelines for care givers to follow. Because psychological, social, psychiatric, and neurologic complications occur frequently, all patients should have early access to social workers (Chapter 16) for planning of physical and financial assistance and referral to local self-help AIDS crisis organizations, as well as psychiatric consultation for monitoring mental status and psychotherapeutic and psychopharmacologic treatment of psychiatric symptoms.

Psychological management requires attention to several key issues. Every health professional should be aware of his or her own possible negative attitudes toward patients with AIDS, fears of caring for the fatally ill, and fears of contagion or prejudices before undertaking patient care. The care giver should not let these attitudes interfere with care. Health professionals should maintain an active and updated file of information about AIDS, its mode of transmission, and cause and treatment, to provide facts and correct misinformation for other staff, friends, and family. New information emerges so rapidly that a poorly informed care giver may misinform a patient.

The care giver must feel comfortable discussing sexual matters with all patients, and know enough about bisexuality and homosexuality to understand the issues and problems as they relate to AIDS transmission. The care giver should be able to evaluate a patient's mental status and identify altered memory, concentration, orientation, and abstraction, and monitor the patient for cognitive dysfunction at each visit. Otherwise, the care giver should have a referral resource regularly available to do the monitoring. Because the central nervous system dysfunction associated with encephalopathy and dementia may precede the definitive AIDS diagnosis, its presence must be assessed along with reactive depression and anxiety.

At time of diagnosis, the care giver must be able to assist the patient in understanding current information about the disease, cause, transmission, available treatment, and sources of care and social support. There must be recognition and discussion of the anxiety and panic associated with fears of progression of the disease, and realistic reassurance given in the context of the situation. Compassionate and sensitive discussion of current treatment and available research protocols must be provided. The range of depressive symptoms (such as sadness, helplessness, hopelessness, and poor self-esteem) should be explored, and questions should be asked about suicidal thoughts and plans. Referrals should be made for support and psychotherapy to deal with loneliness and depression through self-help crisis organizations.

Patients should be encouraged to explore feelings about sexual practices and the sense of guilt that accompanies the knowledge of being a source of contagion to others. Current understanding of precautions for partners, household members, and family, especially "safer sex" with partners, should be discussed, as well as precautions in the use of needles for drug users. Patients should be allowed to express anger toward discrimination, the behavior of others, and stigmatization, and to direct their anger in constructive ways. Help should be offered so they avoid acting in ways that would be self-destructive. Prejudice is likely to interfere with confidentiality and consideration of the patients' emotional well-being.

Fear, uncertainty, and preoccupation with confidentiality are but a few of the many facets of the scientific and societal responses to AIDS. Many deeply troubling issues, particularly the use of the HIV antibody test, tax our abilities to balance the needs of the communities at risk for AIDS and the needs of society as a whole. Sensitivity and respect for the needs of all communities ensure us a responsible and valid solution to these problems. We must avoid, however, the simplistic solutions, such as quarantines, that some propose to protect society.

The acquired immunodeficiency syndrome causes two types of psychosocial crises, one among patients, the other in the general population; both yield opportunities and pitfalls. Medicine and its allied professions can help marshal intelligent responses to regressive societal forces unleashed by the AIDS dilemma, as well as help patients stave off senses of impending doom and hopelessness and accept the losses imposed on them by the disease.

BIBLIOGRAPHY

Allen MH. Primary care of women infected with the human immunodeficiency virus. *Obstet Gynecol Clin North Am.* 1990;17(3):557–569.

Alter MJ, Hadler SC, Margolis HS, et al. The changing epidemiology of hepatitis B in the United States. *JAMA.* 1990;263:1218–1222.

American Academy of Pediatrics. *Report of the common infectious disease.* 22nd ed. Elk Grove, IL: American Academy of Pediatrics; 1991.

American Academy of Pediatrics Task Force on Pediatrics AIDS. Perinatal human immunodeficiency virus (HIV) testing. *AAP News.* 1992;8:20.

Anderson RM, May RM. Understanding the AIDS pandemic. *Sci Am.* 1992;5:58–66.

Baker J, Muma RD. Counseling patients with HIV infection. *Phys Assist.* 1991;15(7):40–42, 47–48.

Barrio JL, Harcup C, Baier HJ, et al. Value of repeat fiberoptic bronchoscopies and significance of nondiagnostic bronchoscopic results in patients with the acquired immunodeficiency syndrome. *Am Rev Respir Dis.* 1987; 135(2):422–425.

Berger JR. Neurologic complications of human immunodeficiency virus infection. *Postgrad Med.* 1987;81:72–79.

Boricic A, Kotler DP. Combating chronic diarrhea in AIDS patients. *Phys Assist.* 1990;14:101–114.

Braun MM, Cauthen G. Relationship of the human immunodeficiency virus epidemic to pediatric tuberculosis and *Bacillus Calmette-Guerin* immunization. *Pediatr Infect Dis J.* 1992;11:220–227.

Broder S, ed. *AIDS: Modern Concepts and Therapeutic Changes.* New York: Marcel Dekker, Inc.; 1987.

Bruhn JG. What to say to persons with HIV disease. *South Med J.* 1991;84:1430–1434.

Burroughs MB, Edelson PJ. Medical care of the HIV infected child. In: Edelson PJ, ed. Childhood AIDS. *Pediatr Clin North Am.* 1991;38:153–167.

Caldwell MB, Rogers MF. Epidemiology of the Pediatric HIV Infection. In: Edelson PJ, ed. Childhood AIDS. *Pediatr Clin North Am.* 1991;38:153–167.

Carney W, Rubin R, Hoffman R, et al. Analysis of T-lymphocyte subsets in cytomegalovirus mononucleosis. *J Immunol.* 1981;126:2114–2116.

Centers for Disease Control. Classification System for Human Immunodeficiency Virus (HIV) Infection in Children Under 13 years of Age. *MMWR.* April 1987: 225–230, 235.

Centers for Disease Control. Classification System for Human T-lymphotropic Virus Type III/Lymphadenopathy-Associated Virus Infections. *MMWR* May 1986: 334–339.

Centers for Disease Control. Guidelines for prophylaxis against *Pneumocystis carinii* pneumonia for children infected with human immunodeficiency virus. *MMWR.* 1991;40:RR-2.

Centers for Disease Control. *HIV/AIDS Surveillance Report.* August 1991:5.

Centers for Disease Control. *HIV/AIDS Surveillance Report.* January 1992:1–22.

Centers for Disease Control. Public health service guidelines for counseling and antibody testing to prevent HIV infection and AIDS. *MMWR.* 1987;36:509–515.

Centers for Disease Control. Interpretation and use of the western blot assay for serodiagnosis of human immunodeficiency virus type-1 infections. *MMWR*. 1989; 38:1–7.

Centers for Disease Control. 1989 sexually transmitted diseases treatment guidelines. *MMWR*. 1989;38:1–43.

Centers for Disease Control. The HIV / AIDS epidemic: the first 10 years. *MMWR*. 1991;40:357.

Centers for Disease Control. Update: Acquired immunodeficiency syndrome—United States, 1981–1991. *MMWR*. 1991;40:358–363, 369.

Centers for Disease Control. The second 100,000 cases of acquired immunodeficiency syndrome—United States. *MMWR*. June 1981–December 1991;41(2):28–29.

Charlottesville AIDS Resource Network. *Safe Sex*. Rockville, MD; 1986.

Chess J, Fisher J. Ophthalmologic manifestations of AIDS. *Phys Assist*. 1989;13:130–135.

Clement M, Franke E, Wisniewski TL. Managing the HIV-positive patient. *Patient Care*. 1989:51–87.

DeVita VT, ed. *AIDS: Etiology, Diagnosis, Treatment and Prevention*. New York: J.B. Lippincott Company; 1985.

De Wolf F, Roos M, Lange JMA, et al. Decline in CD4+ cell numbers reflects increase in HIV-1 replication. *AIDS Resource Human Retroviruses*. 1988;4(6):433–440.

Edelson PJ, ed. Childhood AIDS. *Pediatr Clin North Am*. 1991;38:153–167.

Editorial. Zidovudine for symptomless HIV infection. *Lancet*. 1990;355:821–822.

Ellerbrock TV, Rogers MF. Epidemiology of human immunodeficiency virus infection in women in the United States. *Obstet Gynecol Clin North Am*. 1990;917:523–544.

Fairbanks KD, Sharp V. AIDS Update. *Clinician Rev*. 1992;(2)3:127–138.

Farthing CF, et al. *A Colour Atlas of AIDS*. Ipswich, England: Wolfe Medical Publications Ltd; 1986.

Fischl MA, et al. The efficacy of azidothymidine (AZT) in the treatment of patients with AIDS and AIDS-related complex. *N Engl J Med.* 1987;317:185–191.

Fischl MA, Richman DD, Hansen H, et al. The safety and efficacy of zidovudine (AZT) in the treatment of subjects with mildly symptomatic human immunodeficiency virus type I (HIV) infection: a double-blind, placebo-controlled trial. *Ann Intern Med.* 1990;112:727–737.

Friedman AH. The retinal lesions of the acquired immune deficiency syndrome. *Br Am Ophthalmol.* 1984;82:447–492.

Glatt AE, Chirgwin K, Landesman SH, et al. Current concepts: treatment of infections associated with human immunodeficiency virus. *N Engl J Med.* 1988;318:1439–1445.

Golden JA, Hollander H, Stulbarg MS, et al. Bronchoalveolar lavage as the exclusive diagnostic modality for *Pneumocystis carinii* pneumonia. A prospective study among patients with acquired immunodeficiency syndrome. *Chest.* 1986;90(1):18–22.

Greenspan D, et al. *AIDS and the Mouth.* Copenhagen: Munksgaard; 1990.

Haverkos HW. Assessment of therapy for *Pneumocystis carinii* pneumonia. *Am J Med.* 1984;76:501–508.

Healthy People 2000, DHS, PHS. Superintendent of Document, U.S. Government Printing Office, 1990.

Holmberg SD, Stewart JA, Gerber AR, et al. Prior herpes simplex virus type 2 infection as a risk factor for HIV infection. *JAMA.* February 1988;259(7):1048–1050.

Holmes VF, Fernandez F. HIV and women, current impact and future implications. *Phys Assist.* May 1989:53–57.

Kaplan LD, Wofsy CB, Volberding PA. Treatment of patients with acquired immunodeficiency syndrome and associated manifestations. *JAMA.* 1987;257:1367–1373.

Kaplan MH, Sadick M, McNutt S, et al. Dermatologic findings and manifestations of acquired immunodeficiency syndrome. *J Am Acad Phys Assist.* 1988;1: 91–108.

Kovacs JA, Kovacs A, Polis M, et al. Cryptococcosis in the acquired immunodeficiency syndrome. *Ann Intern Med.* 1985;103:533–538.

Laskin OL, Stahl-Bayliss CM, Kalman CM, et al. Use of ganciclovir to treat serious cytomegalovirus infections in patients with AIDS. *J Infect Dis.* 1987;155: 323–326.

Levine C, Dubler NN. Uncertain risks and bitter realities; the reproductive choices of HIV-infected women. *Milbank Q.* 1990;(68)3:321–351.

Levy RM, Rosenbloom S, Perrett LV. Neuroradiologic findings in AIDS: A review of 200 cases. *Am J Roentgenol.* 1986;147:977–983.

Marchevsky A, Rosen MJ, Chrystal CT, et al. Pulmonary complications of the acquired immunodeficiency syndrome: a clinicopathologic study of 70 cases. *Hum Pathol.* 1985;16:659–670.

McArthur JH, Palenicek JG, Bowersox LL. Human immunodeficiency virus and the nervous system. *Nurs Clin North Am.* 1988;23:823–841.

McDonald JA, Caruso L, Karayiannis P, et al. Diminished responsiveness of male homosexuals chronic hepatitis B virus carriers with HTLV-III antibodies to recombinant alpha-interferon. *Hepatology.* 1987;7:719–723.

Meng TC, Fischl MA, Boota AH, et al. Combination therapy with zidovudine and dideoxycytidine in patients with advanced human immunodeficiency virus infection. *Ann Intern Med.* 1992;116:13–20.

Merigan TC, Skwron G, Bozzette SA, et al. Circulating p24, antigen levels and responses to dideoxycytidine in human immunodeficiency virus (HIV) infections: a phase I and II study. *Ann Intern Med.* 1989;110:189–194.

Meyers A, Weitzman M. Pediatric HIV disease: the newest chronic illness of childhood. In: Edelson PJ, ed. *Childhood AIDS. Pediatr Clin North Am.* 1991;38:153–167.

McKinney RE Jr, Maha MA, Conner EM, et al. and the Protocol 043 Study Group. A multicenter trial of oral zidovudine in children with advanced human immunodeficiency virus disease. *N Engl J Med.* 1991;324: 1018–1025.

Minkoff HL, DeHovitz JA. Care of women infected with the human immunodeficiency virus. *JAMA.* 1991;266 (16):2253–2258.

Mosca JD, Bednarik DP, Raj NBK, et al. Herpes simplex virus type-1 can reactivate transcription of latent human immunodeficiency virus. *Nature.* 1987;325:67–70.

Moss AR, Bacchetti P, Osmond D, et al. Seropositivity for HIV and the development of AIDS or AIDS related condition: three year followup of the San Francisco General Hospital cohort. *Br Med J.* 1988;296:745–750.

Muma RD, Pollard RB. Therapeutics for human immunodeficiency virus infection and associated illnesses. *Phys Assist.* 1992;16(4):21–30.

Muma RD, Borucki MJ, Lyons BA, et al. Evaluation of patients infected with human immunodeficiency virus type I part II: Diagnostic and psychosocial evaluation. *Phys Assist.* 1991;15(2):15,19–22.

Muma RD, Borucki MJ, Lyons BA, et al. Evaluation of patients infected with human immunodeficiency virus type I part I: History and physical evaluation. *Phys Assist.* 1991;15(1):23–32.

Muma RD, Lyons BA, Borucki MJ, et al. AIDS dementia complex: a diagnostic and therapeutic challenge. *J Acad Phys Assist.* 1991;4(2):102–8.

Murphy MF, Metcalfe P, Waters AH, et al. Incidence and mechanism of neutropenia and thrombocytopenia in patients with human immunodeficiency virus infection. *Br J Hematol.* 1987;66:337–340.

Murray JF, Garay SM, Hopewell PC, et al. Pulmonary complications of the acquired immunodeficiency syndrome: an update. Report of the Second National

Heart, Lung, and Blood Institute Workshop. *Am Rev Respir Dis.* 1987;135(2): 504–509.

Nanda D. Human immunodeficiency virus infection in pregnancy. *Obstet Gynecol Clin North Am.* 1990;(17)3: 617–626.

Navia BA, Jordan BD, Price RW. The AIDS dementia complex: I. Clinical Features. *Ann Neurol.* 1986;19: 517–524.

Odajunk C, Muggia FM. Treatment of Kaposi's sarcoma: overview and analysis by clinical setting. *J Clin Oncol.* 1985;3:1277–1285.

OSHA Instruction CPC 2-2-44C. Enforcement procedures for the occupational exposure to bloodborne pathogens standard. March 1992; 29 CFR 1910.1030.

Pitt J. Perinatal human immunodeficiency virus infection in pregnancy. *Obstet Gynecol Clin North Am.* 1990;917: 617–626.

Price RW, Sidtis J, Rosenblum M. The AIDS dementia complex: some current questions. *Ann Neurol.* 1988;23 (suppl):27–33.

Prober CG, Gershon AA. Medical management of newborns and infants born to human immunodeficiency virus-sero-positive mothers. *Pediatr Infect Dis J.* 1991;10:684–694.

Recommendations for preventing transmission of human immunodeficiency virus and hepatitis B virus to patients during exposure-prone invasive producers. *MMWR.* July 1991:1–9.

Recommendations for prevention of HIV transmission in health-care settings. *MMWR.* August 1987:1s–18s.

Revision of the CDC Surveillance Case Definition for Acquired Immunodeficiency Syndrome. *MMWR.* August 1987:1s–15s.

Richman DD, Fischl MA, Grieco MH, et al. The toxicity of azidothymidine (AZT) in the treatment of patients with AIDS and AIDS-related complex: a double-blind, placebo controlled trial. *N Engl J Med.* 1987;317:192–197.

Rogers MF, Chin-Yin O, Kilborne B, et al. Advances and problems in the diagnosis of human immunodeficiency virus infection in infants. *Pediatr Infect Dis J.* 1991;10: 523–531.

Rosenblum ML, ed. *AIDS and the Nervous System.* New York: Raven Press; 1988.

Rothenberg R, Woelfel M, Stoneburner R, et al. Survival with the acquired immunodeficiency syndrome. *N Engl J Med.* 1987;317:1297–1302.

Ruedy J, Schechter M, Montaner JSG. Zidovudine for early human immunodeficiency virus (HIV) infection: who, when, and how? *Ann Intern Med.* 1990;[Editorial]112:721–722.

Rustgi VK, Hoofnagle JH, Gerin JL, et al. Hepatitis B virus infection in the acquired immunodeficiency syndrome. *Ann Intern Med.* 1984;101:795–797.

Sattler FR, Cowan R, Nielsen DM, et al. Trimethoprim sulfamethoxazole compared with pentamidine for treatment of *Pneumocystis carinii* pneumonia in the acquired immunodeficiency syndrome: a prospective, noncrossover study. *Ann Intern Med.* August 1988;109: 280–287.

Schrier R, Rice G, Oldstone M. Suppression of natural killer cell activity and T-cell proliferation by fresh isolates of human cytomegalovirus. *J Infect Dis.* 1986;153: 1084–1091.

Shayne VT, Kaplan BJ. Double victims: poor women and AIDS. *Women & Health.* 1991;(17)1:21–37.

Silverman S Jr. *Color Atlas of Oral Manifestations of AIDS.* Toronto. Philadelphia: BC Decker; 1989.

Smeltzer SC, Whipple B. Women and HIV infection. *Image; J Nurs Sch.* 1991;(23)4:249–255.

Soave R, Johnson WD. Cryptosporidium and isospora infections. *J Infect Dis.* 1988;157:255–299.

Spiegel L, Mayars A. Psychosocial aspects of AIDS in children and adolescents. In: Edelson PJ, ed. *Childhood AIDS. Pediatr Clin North Am.* 1991;38:153–167.

Starke JR. Modern approach to the diagnosis and management of tuberculosis in children. *Pediatr Clin North Am.* 1991;38:153–167.

Statistics from the Centers for Disease Control. *AIDS.* 1992;6(13)343–345.

Statistics from the World Health Organization and the Centers for Disease Control. *AIDS.* 1992;6:753–757.

Suttmann U, Willers H, Gerdelmann R, et al. Cytomegalovirus infection in HIV-1-infected individuals. *Infection.* 1988;16(2):111–114.

Terrance Higgins Trust, Ltd. AIDS and HIV Medical Briefing. Rev. ed., 1987.

Volberding PA, Lagakos SW, Koch MA, et al. Zidovudine in asymptomatic human immunodeficiency virus infection. A controlled trial in persons with fewer than 500 CD4-positive cells per cubic millimeter. *N Engl J Med.* 1990;322:941–949.

Wharton MJ, Coleman DL, Wofsy C, et al. Trimethoprim-sulfamethoxazole or pentamidine for *Pneumocystis carinii* pneumonia in the acquired immunodeficiency syndrome. *Ann Intern Med.* 1986;105:37–44.

Wormser GP, ed. *AIDS and Other Manifestations of HIV Infection.* Park Ridge, NJ: Noyes Publications; 1987.

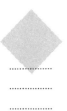

INDEX

The page numbers for entries appearing in boxes are followed by a b; those for entries appearing in figure captions, by an f; and those for entries appearing in tables, by a t.

Abdomen, examination of, 163-164

Absolute granulocyte count, 108, 109, 118

Absolute T4 (CD4) cell count, 167
  laboratory data on, 113–116
  pediatric HIV and, 178, 179t, 180
  PGL and, 43

Abstinence, 246

Acceptance, 224

Acute hepatitis, 81, 82

Acyclovir, 102t, 107, 120t, 124, 125

Adaptation, psychological, 261–264

ADC, *see* AIDS dementia complex

Adenoids, 23

Adolescents, 182
  CMV in, 64
  epidemiology of disease in, 7, 8, 11, 13
  grief stages in, 225
  psychosocial aspects of disease in, 197–198

Adriamycin, 134

Adverse drug reactions, 99–109, 112, 116, 119, 120, 156b
  of acyclovir, 102t, 107, 119t
  of aminoglycosides, 119t
  of amphotericin B, 50, 57–58, 102t, 107, 118, 119t
  of atovaquone, 49
  of ciprofloxacin, 102t
  of clarithromycin, 102t
  of clotrimazole, 67
  of co-trimoxazole, 102t
  of dapsone, 102t, 104
  of ddC, 36, 103t, 104, 105, 121
  of ddI, 36–37, 102t, 104, 105, 121
  defined, 100
  of ethambutol, 102t
  of ethionamide, 104
  of fluconazole, 58, 67, 102t, 121
  of flucytosine, 102t, 108, 119t
  of foscarnet, 65–66, 102t, 107, 119t
  of ganciclovir, 65, 102t, 105, 108, 119t
  of interferon, 83
  of isoniazid, 53, 102t, 104, 121

Adverse drug reactions (*cont.*)
of itraconazole, 51, 103t, 121
of ketoconazole, 67, 103t, 118, 121, 143
management of, 103, 105, 106, 107–108, 109
of metronidazole, 103t, 104
of pentamidine, 48–49, 103t, 105, 107, 108, 119t, 121
of pyrazinamide, 53, 103t, 121
of pyrimethamine, 55, 103t, 108, 118
recognition of, 100–103, 104, 106, 107, 108
of ribavirin, 186
of rifampin, 53, 103t, 119t, 121
of sulfadiazine, 55, 103t, 107
of sulfa drugs, 119t
of sulfonamides, 108
of TMP-SMX, 48, 118, 121, 183
of ZDV, 36, 103t, 108, 197
AFB smear, 170
Africa, 7, 8, 9, 78
African-Americans, 146
epidemiology of disease in, 11
focal segmental glomerulosclerosis in, 120
prevention in, 252, 253–254, 255, 256
Age, 10
AIDS dementia complex (ADC), 13, 60–61, 63f
clinical manifestations of, 61, 62t
diagnosis of, 61
laboratory data on, 170
pediatric HIV and, 198
in physical examination, 161–162
psychosocial aspects of, 268
treatment of, 61
AIDS-related complex, 36
Alaskan natives, 11
Albumin, 116
Alcohol use, 28, 30, 32, 106, 120, 121

Alkaline phosphatase, 79, 121
Allergic reactions, 17, 100
Alopecia, 132
ALT, 120
American Indians, *see* Native Americans
Amikacin, 52, 71
Aminoglycosides, 52, 120t, *see also specific types*
Amitriptyline, 105, 125
Amoebiasis, 158
Amphotericin B
adverse reactions of, 50, 57–58, 102t, 107, 118, 120t
for cryptococcal meningitis, 57–58
for cryptococcosis, 128
for histoplasmosis, 50, 129
Amylase, 106, 122
Anal intercourse, 9, 244, 245, 246, 254
Anaphylaxis, 17
Anemia, 36, 112, 166, 186, 197
histoplasmosis and, 49, 117
laboratory data on, 116–117
macrocytic, 117t
megaloblastic, 36, 55
microcytic, 116, 117t
normochromic, 116
normocytic, 116, 117t
pregnancy and, 144
Anergy, 19
Anger, 224, 225, 265
Anilingus, 9
Anorexia, 156b
Antibiotics, 125, 143, *see also specific types*
Antibodies, 15, 24, 246
in congenital syphilis, 187, 192
in hepatitis, 80, 82
laboratory data on, 113
pediatric HIV and, 180, 181
Antigen-presenting cells, 16, 18
Antigens, 15–16, 18, 19
cardiolipin-lecithin, 95

cryptococcal, 57, 168
    hepatitis, 82, 84
    laboratory data on, 112
    p24, *see* p24 antigens
    surface, 80, 81, 82, 251, 252
Antigen skin testing, 52
Antihistamines, 130, 131, 132
Anxiety, 221–223, 265, 268, 269
Aphasia, 58
Aphthous ulcers, 159
Argyll-Robertson pupils, 91
Arthritis, syphilitic, 90
Ascites, 120, 163, 164
Aseptic meningitis, 154, 155, 162
Asian Americans, 11, 252
AST, 120
Asymptomatic patients, 165–166
    pediatric, 199t
Ataxias, 91
Athlete's foot, 127–128
Atovaquone, 47–48, 49
Atypical mycobacteriosis, 12,
    162
Autologous blood transfusions,
    247
AZT, *see* Zidovudine

B cells, 16, 17, 180, 193
B19 parvovirus, 117
Bacterial endocarditis, 163
Bacterial folliculitis, 130
Bacterial infections, 163, 170, *see
    also specific types*
    dental, 214t
    immunology and, 16
    pediatric HIV and, 178
Bacterial pneumonia, 154
Bargaining, 224
Barium enemas, 170
Beta 2 Microglobulin (B2M),
    116, 167
Bilirubin, 121
    hepatitis and, 79, 80, 120
    pregnancy and, 143–144
Biopsies

bone marrow, 168
brain, 54
    CNS toxoplasmosis in, 54
    hepatitis in, 81, 83
    KS in, 133
    lung, 47, 182–183
    M. tuberculosis in, 52
    MAC in, 70
    molluscum contagiosum in,
        126
    outpatient nursing and, 234, 241
    PCP in, 47
    pediatric PCP in, 182–183
    primary brain lymphoma in, 59
    syphilis in, 92
    transbronchial, 169
Bisexuals, 2
    counseling of, 28
    epidemiology of disease in, 8, 11
    in minority groups, 254–255
    psychosocial issues for, 263, 268
Blacks, *see* African-Americans
Blastomycosis, 168
Bleach, 249
Bleomycin, 134
Blindness, 64
Blood-borne transmission, 9,
    23, 243–244, *see also specific
    modes of*
    of CMV, 64
    of HBV, 78
Blood clotting factors, 9, 246,
    247
Blood donation, 248
Blood products, 9, 10, 244
    CMV in, 64
    HBV in, 78
    prevention of infection via,
        246–247
Blood transfusions, 10, 11, 137
    autologous, 247
    hepatitis and, 78
    outpatient nursing and, 234,
        236, 240b, 241
    pediatric HIV and, 177

Blood transfusions (*cont.*)
  prevention of infection via,
    246–247
  psychosocial aspects of
    infection via, 263
B2M, *see* Beta 2 Microglobulin
Bone marrow, 117, 243
Bone marrow aspiration, 234,
  241
Bone marrow biopsies, 168
Bone marrow suppression, 108,
  109, 117
Brain biopsies, 54
Brain tissue, 243
Breast feeding, 137, 144, 177,
  180, 243, 247
Bronchiolitis, 185
Bronchoalveolar lavage, 47, 169
Bronchodilators, 184
Bronchoscopy, 47, 52, 169, 170,
  182
Brudzinski's sign, 161

California, 2, 11
Campylobacter, 154, 170
Cancer, 21, 56, *see also specific
  types*
Candida albicans, 66
Candidiasis
  dermatologic manifestations of,
    127
  esophageal, 12, 66–67, 140
  hairy leukoplakia and, 215
  immunology and, 18
  mucocutaneous, 178
  oral, *see* Oral candidiasis
  in physical examination, 160
  rectal, 154
  vaginal, 138, 142–143, 154
Capreomycin, 52
Cardiolipin-lecithin antigens, 95
Cardiomyopathy, 159, 163
Care givers, 266–267, 268–269
Casual contact, 10, 243
Catheters, 234–236

  dressing changes and, 237–239b
  flushing and rinsing of,
    232–233b
  injection cap changing in, 233b
CD2 (T3) cells, 17
CD4 cells, *see* T4 (CD4) cells
CD8 cells, *see* T8 (CD8) cells
CDC, *see* Centers for Disease
  Control and Prevention
Cefoxitin, 142
Ceftriaxone, 95t, 140
Cell-mediated immunity, 15, 17,
  18, 38
Center for Substance Abuse
  Treatment, 212
Centers for Disease Control and
  Prevention (CDC) AIDS
  Education Center, 258
Centers for Disease Control and
  Prevention (CDC) National
  Sexually Transmitted
  Diseases Hotline, 212
Centers for Disease Control and
  Prevention (CDC)
  surveillance case
  definition/classification, 2,
  150
  ADC in, 61
  for adults/adolescents, 13t, 13
  congenital syphilis in, 187,
    189–190b
  hairy leukoplakia in, 215
  HSV in, 216
  of pediatric HIV, 178t
  PGL in, 42
  revised, 151t
  for women, 146
Central nervous system (CNS),
  262, 268
  examination of, 154, 155,
    161–162
  pediatric HIV and, 197
  syphilis and, 93
Central nervous system (CNS)
  cryptococcus, 54

Central nervous system (CNS)
toxoplasmosis, 53–55, 162
Cephalexin, 132
Cerebrospinal fluid (CSF), 9,
139, 166, 243, *see also*
Venereal Disease Research
Laboratory (VDRL)
cryptococcal meningitis in,
56–57
primary brain lymphoma in, 60
syphilis in, 92–95, 141, 187, 191,
193, 194–195
ZDV and, 196
Cervical carcinoma, 13, 140
Cervical cultures, 139
Cervical dysplasia, 138,
140
Cesarean sections, 177
Chancroid, 140–142, 153
Chemotaxis, 19, 108
Chemotherapy, 60, 134, 150
Chest x-rays, 47, 168–169, 182,
184, 185
Chickenpox, 124–125, 197
Children, 15, 43, 78, *see also*
Pediatric human
immunodeficiency virus
Chills, 154
Chlamydia, 139, 142, 166
Cholesterol levels, 116
Chorioretinitis, 54
Chronic active hepatitis, 80
Chronic hepatitis, 79–81, 82,
83–84
Chronic persistent hepatitis, 80
Chronic pulmonary
histoplasmosis, 50
Ciprofloxacin, 52, 70, 102t, 140
Cirrhosis, 77, 80, 81
Clarithromycin, 70, 71, 102t
Clindamycin, 55, 132
Clinical manifestations
of ADC, 61, 62t
of CMV, 64
of CNS toxoplasmosis, 53–54

of cryptococcal meningitis, 56
of *Cryptosporidium,* 68
of esophageal candidiasis, 66
of hepatitis, 79–81
of histoplasmosis, 49
of *M. tuberculosis,* 51
of MAC, 69–70
of oral candidiasis, 66
of PCP, 44–47
of PGL, 42
of primary brain lymphoma,
58–59
of syphilis, 87–88, 89–91
Clinical trials, 212
Clofazimine, 70, 102t
Clotrimazole, 66, 67, 127, 142
CMV, *see* Cytomegalovirus
CNS, *see* Central nervous
system
Coal tar, 130
Coccidioidomycosis, 126, 162,
168
Cold sores, 216
Colitis, 70, 164
CMV, 64, 116
pseudomembranous, 158
Colposcopy, 140
Coma, 53
Communication
cultural barriers to, 257–258
in nursing assessment, 219–220
Community resources, 211–212
Computerized tomography
(CT), 54, 59, 168, 170
Condoms, 145, 146, 245, 246
Condyloma, 126–127, 138, 140,
153, 154, 160, 164
Condylomata lata, 187
Congenital syphilis, 186–195
Conjuctivitis, 186
Contraceptives, 31, 145, 247, *see
also specific types*
Corticosteroids, 47, 130, 131
Co-trimoxazole, 102t
Cotton wool spots, 159, 160

Cough, 158, 185
Counseling, 27–32
    posttest, 25, 27, 30–32
    pretest, 27–28, 29–30
Creatinine, 107, 108
Crotamiton, 133
Cryotherapy, 126, 127
Cryptococcal antigens, 57, 168
Cryptococcal meningitis, 55–58,
    155, 162
Cryptococcosis, 126, 128, 162
Cryptococcus, 12, 43, 54, 160, 168
Cryptococcus neoformans, 18, 56
Cryptosporidiosis, 12, 121, 158,
    170
Cryptosporidium, 1, 18, 67–68
CSF, *see* Cerebrospinal fluid
CT, *see* Computerized
    tomography
Cultural differences, 257–258
Cunnilingus, 9
Curettage, 126
Cycloserine, 70–71
Cytomegalovirus (CMV), 43,
    62–66
    clinical manifestations of, 64
    CNS toxoplasmosis confused
        with, 54
    diagnosis of, 65
    epidemiology of, 12
    hepatic dysfunction and, 64, 121
    immunology and, 18
    KS and, 133
    laboratory data on, 167, 169
    pancreatic dysfunction and, 122
    pancreatitis and, 105
    peripheral neuropathy and, 104
    in physical examination, 162,
        163
    syphilis confused with, 93
    treatment of, 65–66
Cytomegalovirus (CMV) colitis,
    64, 116
Cytomegalovirus (CMV)
    esophagitis, 64

Cytomegalovirus (CMV)
    pneumonia, 44, 64
Cytomegalovirus (CMV)
    retinitis, 64, 65, 160, 236
Cytotoxicity, 19
Cytotoxic T cells, 15, 17, 81
Cytovene, *see* Ganciclovir

Dapsone, 102t, 104, 196t
ddC, *see* Zalcitabine
ddI, *see* Didanosine
Debility, 156b
Delayed hypersensitivity, 18
Delivery, transmission during,
    10, 137, 144, 177, 244
Dementia, *see* AIDS dementia
    complex
Demographics, 10–11
Denial, 208, 224
Dentistry, 213–216, 250, 251
Depo-Provera, 145
Depression, psychological, 198,
    205, 224, 266, 268, 269
Dermatologic manifestations,
    123–134
    infectious, 123, 124–129
    neoplastic, 123, 133–134
    non-infectious, 123, 129–133
Developmental stages, 225
DHPG, *see* Ganciclovir
Diabetes, 121
Diagnosis
    of ADC, 61
    of CMV, 65
    of CNS toxoplasmosis, 54
    of cryptococcal meningitis,
        56–57
    of *Cryptosporidium,* 68
    of esophageal candidiasis, 66
    of hepatitis, 82
    of histoplasmosis, 50
    laboratory data in, 112–113,
        164–170
    of *M. tuberculosis,* 52
    of MAC, 70

of oral candidiasis, 66
of PCP, 47
of pediatric HIV, 177–178
of PGL, 42
of primary brain lymphoma,
    59–60
of syphilis, 91–95
in women, 138
Diaphragms, 145
Diarrhea, 1, 36, 41, 155, 157b,
    158, 170
    abdominal symptoms caused
        by, 164
    Cryptosporidium and, 68
    hyponatremia and, 119
    MAC and, 69, 70
    medical history of, 154
    traveler's, 158
Didanosine (ddI), 36–37, 102t,
    104, 105, 121
Diffuse hepatitis, 120
Diplopia, 155, 157b
Discrimination, 263
Disseminated histoplasmosis,
    50
Distress, psychological, 264–266
District of Columbia, 2, 11
DNA, 21, 25, 180, 181
DNA polymerase, 81
DNA probes, 52, 70, 112
Doxycycline, 142
Drug abuse, 27–28, 32, 146, 209,
    see also Injecting drug users
Dysarthria, 155
Dysphagia, 157b
Dyspnea, 157b, 158

EBV, *see* Epstein-Barr virus
Electrocautery, 127
Electrocoagulation, 126
Electrodesiccation, 126
Electroencephalography (EEG),
    170
ELISA, *see* Enzyme-linked
    immunosorbent assay

Encephalitis, 91, 155, 162, 168
Encephalopathy, 196, 268
Endocarditis, 163
Entamoeba histolytica, 154
Envelope glycoproteins, 24, 25,
    113
Enzyme immunoassay, 166
Enzyme-linked immunosorbent
    assay (ELISA), 25, 113
Eosinophilic pustular
    folliculitis (EPF), 130–131
EPF, *see* Eosinophilic pustular
    folliculitis
Epidemiology, 7–13
    demographic characteristics in,
        10–11
    of diseases associated with
        AIDS, 11–12
    geographic distribution in, 11
    of hepatitis, 78–79
    in minority groups, 11, 253–254
    of pediatric HIV, 7, 11, 13, 177
    of transmission, 7–10
    in women, 8, 11, 137
Epstein-Barr virus (EBV), 43,
    163
Erikson, Erik, 225
Escherichia coli, 170
Esophageal candidiasis, 12,
    66–67, 140
Esophagitis, 64
Ethambutol, 52, 71, 102t
Ethionamide, 104
Etiology, 21–25
Evaluation, 149–171
    laboratory data in, 164–170
    patient history in, 152–154
    physical examination in,
        159–164
    psychosocial, 170–171
    by social workers, 204–207
    systems review in, 154–159
Eyes, examination of, 159–160

Fatigue, 154

Feces, CMV in, 64
Fellatio, 9
Fever, 154, 156b, 159, 168, 185
Fialuridine, 83
Filgrastim, 102t, 109
Fisting, 9
Florida, 11
Fluconazole
  adverse reactions of, 58, 67,
    102t, 121
  for candidiasis, 67, 127, 142
  for cryptococcal meningitis, 57,
    58
  for cryptococcosis, 128
  for tinea, 128
Flucytosine, 57, 102t, 108, 120t
Fluorescent treponema
    antibody absorption (FTA
    ABS) test, 166, 187, 191, 194
Fluoroquinolones, 140
Focal segmental
    glomerulosclerosis, 120
Folate, 117
Folinic acid, 55
Folliculitis, 154, 160
  eosinophilic pustular, 130–131
Foscarnet, 65–66, 102t, 107, 120t
France, 23–24
FTA ABS test, see Fluorescent
    treponema antibody
    absorption test
Fungal immunodiffusion, 168
Fungal infections, 154, 159, 163,
    see also specific types
  dental manifestations of, 214t
  dermatologic manifestations of,
    127–129
  pancreatic dysfunction and, 122
  systemic, 128–129
Furosemide, 236

GAG proteins, 24, 25, 38, 113
Gallo, Robert C., 23
Ganciclovir (DHPG), 65, 102t,
    105, 108, 120t

Gastrointestinal system, 64
  examination of, 154, 155, 158
Gay Men's Health Crisis
    hotline, 212
Gender, see Women
Generalized lymphadenopathy,
    118, 178
  persistent, 41, 42–43
Genitalia, examination of, 164
Genital ulcers, 138, 141
Genital warts, see Condyloma
Genitorectal herpes, 154
Genitourinary system,
    examination of, 154
Geographic distribution, 11
Giardia lamblia, 154
Gingivitis, 214, 216
Gonorrhea, 139, 142, 153, 166,
    186
gp 120, 24, 113
gp 160, 113
Granulocytopenia, 36, 117–118
Granulomatous hepatitis,
    120–121
Grasp reflex, 161
Grief stages, 224–225
Griseofulvin, 127
Groshong catheters, 234

Hair changes, 132
Hairy leukoplakia, 159, 214, 215
Haiti/Haitians, 7, 9, 51, 263
HAV, see Hepatitis A virus
HBV, see Hepatitis B virus
HCV, see Hepatitis C virus
HDV, see Hepatitis delta virus
Headaches, 155, 156b, 168
Health care workers, see also
    specific types
  hepatitis in, 78, 249, 251
  prevention of infection in, 244,
    247–252
  transmission of infection to, 10
Heart, examination of, 163
Helper T cells, see T4 (CD4) cells

Hematocrit, 43, 112
Hematologic studies, 116–119
Hematopoiesis, 116
Hematopoietic toxicity, 36
Hemiparesis, 58, 91
Hemoglobin, 43, 112
Hemophiliacs
  epidemiology of infection in, 10
  hepatitis in, 78
  pediatric HIV in, 177
  prevention of infection in, 246
  psychosocial issues for, 263
Hepatic dysfunction, 36–37, 143
  CMV and, 64, 121
  laboratory data on, 120–121
Hepatic failure, 77
Hepatic transaminases, 79, 80,
    82, 83, 84, 166, 167
Hepatitis, 77–84, *see also* specfic
    virus types
  acute, 81, 82
  chronic, 79–81, 82, 83–84
  chronic active, 80
  chronic persistent, 80
  clinical manifestations of, 79–81
  diagnosis of, 82
  diffuse, 120
  epidemiology of, 78–79
  granulomatous, 120–121
  in health care workers, 78, 249,
    251
  laboratory data on, 166, 167
  in physical examination, 164
  syphilitic, 90
  treatment of, 82–84
Hepatitis A virus (HAV), 77, 78,
    82, 166
Hepatitis B surface antigens, 80,
    81, 82, 251, 252
Hepatitis B virus (HBV), 43, 77,
    84, 120, 251, 267
  acute, 81
  chronic, 79–81, 83
  epidemiology of, 78
  etiology/pathogenesis of, 23

  laboratory data on, 166
  medical history of, 153
  pediatric, 186
Hepatitis C virus (HCV), 77, 82,
    84, 120
  chronic, 83–84
  epidemiology of, 78
  laboratory data on, 166
Hepatitis delta virus (HDV), 77,
    78, 81, 82, 84
Hepatitis E virus (HEV), 77, 79,
    82
Hepatomegaly, 70
Hepatosplenomegaly, 49,
    163–164, 178
Hepatotoxicity, 121
Herpes, *see also specific types*
  genitorectal, 154
  immunology and, 18
  medical history of, 153
  perianal, 1
  in physical examination, 164
Herpes encephalitis, 155, 162
Herpes labialis, 216
Herpes simplex virus (HSV),
    125
  dentistry and, 214, 216
  epidemiology of, 12
  laboratory data on, 166, 167
  in physical examination, 159,
    160, 161
  in women, 138, 140, 141
Heterosexual transmission, 8, 9,
    11, 137, 252
HEV, *see* Hepatitis E virus
Hickman catheters, 234
High risk behaviors, 9–10
High risk groups, 165–166
Hispanics, 146
  epidemiology in, 11
  prevention in, 252, 254–255,
    256, 257
Histoplasma, 18
Histoplasma capsulatum, 49
Histoplasmosis, 43, 49–51, 129

Histoplasmosis (*cont.*)
  anemia and, 49, 117
  chronic pulmonary, 50
  clinical manifestations of, 49
  CNS toxoplasmosis confused
    with, 54
  diagnosis of, 50
  disseminated, 50
  laboratory data on, 168, 169
  molluscum contagiosum
    confused with, 126
  in physical examination, 159,
    162
  treatment of, 50–51
HIV, *see* Human
    immunodeficiency virus
Hohn Central Venous Catheter,
    230–231b, 234–236
Homophobia, 261, 267
Homosexuals, 1, 2, 3, 153
  counseling of, 28
  epidemiology of disease in, 8, 11
  hepatitis in, 78
  in minority groups, 253, 254–255
  PGL in, 42
  prevention of infection in, 245,
    246
  psychosocial issues for, 263,
    264, 268
Hospice Link, 212
HPV, *see* Human papilloma
    virus
HSV, *see* Herpes simplex virus
Human immunodeficiency
    virus-2 (HIV-2), 24
Human immunodeficiency
    virus (HIV) dementia, *see*
    AIDS dementia complex
Human immunodeficiency
    virus (HIV) test, 25
  for children, 180–182
  false-negative results on, 30
  false-positive results on, 113
  indeterminate results on, 30, 113

  mandatory, for health care
    workers, 252
  negative results on, 30–31
  positive results on, 30, 31–32,
    113
  psychosocial aspects of, 269
  for women, 138
Human immunodeficiency
    virus (HIV) wasting
    syndrome, 13
Human papilloma virus (HPV),
    126–127, 138, 140
Humoral immunity, 15, 18, 38
Hydrocephalus, 56
Hydrocortisone cream, 129
Hypergammaglobulinemia,
    180, 193
Hypersensitivity reactions, 100,
    103
Hypertriglyceridemia, 106
Hypocalcemia, 106, 111
Hypochondria, 265
Hypoglycemia, 121, 155, 183
Hyponatremia, 107, 119–120
Hypoxia, 155, 169, 170, 184

Ibuprofen, 105
Idiopathic CD4 T
    lymphocytopenia, 18
IDUs, *see* Injecting drug users
Ig, *see* Immunoglobulin
Imipramine, 125
Immediate hypersensitivity, 17
Immigrants, 263
Immune thrombocytopenic
    purpura (ITP), 118
Immunizations, *see* Vaccinations
Immunoglobulin (Ig), 16, 19,
    119, *see also specific types*
Immunoglobulin A (IgA), 16,
    17, 180, 181–182
Immunoglobulin D (IgD), 16
Immunoglobulin E (IgE), 16, 17
Immunoglobulin G (IgG), 16,
    17, 82, 180, 181, 187

Immunoglobulin M (IgM), 16, 17, 82, 181, 187, 191
Immunology, 15–20
Incidence
  of AIDS, 2, 7
  of *M. tuberculosis,* 51
  of PCP, 43
Incontinence, 91, 161
Infectious dermatologic manifestations, 123, 124–129
Inguinal lymphadenopathy, 141
Injecting drug users (IDUs), 2, 137, 153, 243, 244
  counseling of, 28, 29, 30
  epidemiology of disease in, 8, 10, 11
  focal segmental glomerulosclerosis in, 120
  heart problems in, 163
  hepatitis in, 78
  M. tuberculosis in, 51
  in minority groups, 253
  prevention of infection in, 245–246
  psychosocial issues for, 263, 264, 267, 269
  social worker evaluation of, 207
Integrase, 25, 38
Interferons, 16, 77, 83, 84
Interleukins, 16
Interstitial pneumonia, 178
  lymphoid, 163, 182, 184
Intrauterine device (IUD), 145
In utero transmission, 10, 244
In vitro production assays, 181, 182
Iron deficiencies, 116
Isoniazid, 52, 53, 102t, 104, 121, 185
Isosporiasis, 158
Italy, 78
ITP, *see* Immune thrombocytopenic purpura
Itraconazole, 50, 51, 103t, 121, 129

Jaundice, 49, 79, 120, 121
Jock itch, 128

Kanamycin, 52
Kaposi's sarcoma (KS), 1, 123, 133–134, 159
  anemia and, 116
  CNS toxoplasmosis confused with, 54
  epidemiology of, 12
  pancreatic dysfunction and, 122
  in physical examination, 159, 160, 163, 164
  psychosocial aspects of, 262
  pulmonary, 44
Keratolytics, 126
Kernicterus, 144
Kernig's sign, 161
Ketoconazole, 67, 103t, 118, 121, 142
Killer cells, 19
KS, *see* Kaposi's sarcoma
Kübler-Ross, Elisabeth, 224

Laboratory data, 111–122
  diagnosis established with, 112–113, 164–170
  on hematologic abnormalities, 116–119
  on hepatic dysfunction, 120–121
  on pancreatic dysfunction, 121–122
  on pediatric HIV, 178–180
  on renal dysfunction, 119–120
Laser surgery, 126, 127
Lasix, 236
Latency period of infection, 23
Latent syphilis, 88, 153
  clinical manifestations of, 89–90
  diagnosis of, 92, 93–94
  treatment of, 95t
Lentiviruses, 22
Leukemia, 43
Leukocytes, 133

Leukocytosis, 142
Leukopenia, 49
Lindane lotion, 133
LIP, *see* Lymphoid interstitial
    pneumonia
Lipase, 121, 122
Lomotil, 68
Low risk behaviors, 10
Lumbar punctures, 234, 241
Lung biopsies, 47, 182–183
Lungs, *see entries under*
    Pulmonary
Lymphadenopathy, 157b
    generalized, *see* Generalized
        lymphadenopathy
    histoplasmosis and, 49
    inguinal, 141
    MAC and, 70
    pediatric tuberculosis and, 185
    syphilis and, 88
Lymph nodes, 23, 163, 243
Lymphocytes, 19, 184, *see also*
    specific types
Lymphoid interstitial
    pneumonia (LIP), 163, 182,
    184
Lymphokines, 19, *see also*
    specific types
Lymphoma
    anemia and, 116
    CNS toxoplasmosis confused
        with, 54
    non-Hodgkin's, 1, 155, 159
    in physical examination, 162,
        164
    primary brain, 58–60, 162
    syphilis and, 93

MAC, *see Mycobacterium avium*
    complex
Macrocytic anemia, 117t
Macrophages, 16, 18, 70, 184
Magnetic resonance imaging
    (MRI), 54, 93
Mammograms, 140

Maternal transmission, 247, *see*
    also Pregnancy
    breast-feeding and, 137, 144,
        177, 180, 243, 247
    at delivery, 10, 137, 144, 177, 244
    epidemiology of, 10
    in utero, 10, 244
    neonatal, 253
    pathogenesis of, 23
    perinatal, 9, 177
    placental, *see* Placental
        transmission
    postpartum, 244
Measles, 197
Medical history, 153–154
Mediterranean area, 78
Megaloblastic anemia, 36, 55
Meningitis, 91
    aseptic, 154, 155, 162
    cryptococcal, 55–58, 155, 162
    tuberculosis, 155
Methotrexate, 130
Metronidazole, 103t, 104
Microcephaly, 197
Microcytic anemia, 116, 117t
Middle East, 78
Military service personnel, 264
Minority groups, 11, 252–258,
    see also specific groups
Mississippi River Valley, 49
Mites, 132
Molluscum contagiosum, 126,
    128, 154
Monocytes, 16, 18
Mononucleosis, 62–64
Montagnier, Luc, 23
Mosquitos, 10
Mouth, examination of, 159
Mouth-to-mouth resuscitation,
    248–249
MRI, *see* Magnetic resonance
    imaging
Mucocutaneous candidiasis, 178
Multiple sexual partners, 244,
    245

Mycobacterioses, 18, 158, 159
  atypical, 12, 162
  laboratory data on, 170
  in physical examination, 162, 163, 164
  syphilis confused with, 93
Mycobacterium avium, 69, 117
Mycobacterium avium complex (MAC), 69–71
Mycobacterium avium-intracellulare, 1, 69, 70, 160
Mycobacterium kansasii, 117
Mycobacterium scrofulaceum, 69
Mycobacterium tuberculosis, 51–53, 70, 166

Naftifine, 127
National AIDS Clearinghouse, 212
National AIDS Hotline, 212
National Institutes of Health AIDS Education Center, 258
Native Americans, 11, 252, 257
Necrotizing gingivitis, 214, 216
Needle exchange programs, 253
Needle sharing, 10, 29, 32, 243, 245, 269
Neisseria gonorrhea, 166
Neonatal transmission, 253
Neoplasms, 162, 163
  dental manifestations of, 214t
  dermatologic manifestations of, 123, 133–134
  epidemiology of, 8
Nephrotoxicity, 119–120, 120t
Neurologic disturbances, dental manifestations of, 214t
Neuropathies
  peripheral, 36, 103, 104–105
  poly-, 162
  sensory, 162
Neurosyphilis, 153, 193

clinical manifestations of, 90–91
diagnosis of, 92–95
laboratory data on, 166
in physical examination, 162
treatment of, 95t
Neutropenia, 103, 108–109, 166, 197
New Jersey, 11
New York, 1, 2, 11
Night sweats, 154, 156b, 185
Nocardiosis, 54, 154
Non-Hodgkin's lymphoma, 1, 155, 159
Non-infectious dermatologic manifestations, 123, 129–133
Nonoxinol-9, 246
Nonsteroidal antiinflammatory drugs, 120t
Nontransforming retroviruses, 22
Nontreponemal assays, 94t
Normochromic anemia, 116
Normocytic anemia, 116, 117t
Norplant, 145
Nortriptyline, 105
Nucleoside analogues, 36–37, *see also specific types*
Nursing assessment, 217–226, *see also* Outpatient nursing
  communication in, 219–220
  of grief stages, 224–225
  psychosocial, 223
  of self, 218
Nutrition, 183–184
Nystatin, 127

Occupational transmission, 10
Ofloxacin, 52
Ohio River Valley, 49
OKT3 cells, 17
OKT4 cells, *see* T4 (CD4) cells
OKT8 cells, *see* T8 (CD8) cells
Onycholysis, 160

Onychomycosis, 127, 128
Opportunistic infections, 3, 5, 8, 13, 19, 36, 92, *see also specific types*
Oral candidiasis, 66–67, 154
  clinical manifestations of, 66
  dentistry and, 214, 215
  diagnosis of, 66
  in physical examination, 159
  treatment of, 66–67
Oral contraceptives, 143, 145
Oral sex, 245
Organ transplantation, 16, 18, 56
Osteochondritis, 187
Outpatient nursing, 229–242, *see also* Nursing assessment
  blood transfusions and, 234, 236, 240b, 241
  catheter care and, *see* Catheters
  patient education and, 242

p6 protein, 38
p9 protein, 38
p15 protein, 38, 113
p17 protein, 38, 113
p24 antigen, 24, 36, 38
  laboratory data on, 113, 116
  pediatric HIV and, 180, 181, 182
  ZDV and, 196
Pacific Islanders, 11, 252, 257
Pancreatic dysfunction, 121–122
Pancreatitis, 36, 103, 105–106, 122, 183
Panic attacks, 265, 269
Pap smears, 139, 140
Paraparesis, 161
Parasitic infections, 16, 19, 159, 170, *see also specific types*
Paronychia, 127, 160
Parotitis, 178
Partial thromboplastin time, 118–119
Pathogenesis, 21–25
Patient education, 170–171, 242
Patient history, 152–154

PCP, *see Pneumocystis carinii* pneumonia
PCR, *see* Polymerase chain reaction
Pediatric human immunodeficiency virus (HIV), 2, 3, 43, 177–200, *see also* Maternal transmission; Pregnancy
  diagnosis of, 177–178
  epidemiology of, 7, 11, 13, 177
  infectious complications in, 182–186
  laboratory evaluation of, 178–180
  in minority groups, 252
  prevention of, 244
  psychosocial aspects of, 197–198, 263, 264
  syphilis and, 186–195
  testing for, 180–182
  vaccinations and, 197, 198t
  ZDV for, 180, 195–197
Pelvic inflammatory disease, 138, 141–142, 145
Penicillin, 95t, 141, 193, 194
Pentamidine, 47, 169, 183, 196t
  adverse reactions of, 48–49, 103t, 105, 107, 108, 120t, 121
  pregnancy and, 143, 144
Perianal herpes, 1
Perinatal transmission, 9, 177
Periodontitis, 214, 216
Periostitis, 187
Peripheral nervous system, 161–162
Peripheral neuropathies, 36, 103, 104–105
Persistent generalized lymphadenopathy (PGL), 41, 42–43
Personal protective equipment (PPE), 247–248
PGL, *see* Persistent generalized lymphadenopathy

Phenytoin, 125
Phlebotomy, 248
Physical examination, 159–164
Placental transmission, 144, 177
  of syphilis, 187
Platelets, 43, 118
Pneumocystis carinii pneumonia
  (PCP), 1, 43–49, 121, 167
  clinical manifestations of, 44–47
  diagnosis of, 47
  epidemiology of, 11
  immunology and, 18
  laboratory data on, 169
  pediatric HIV and, 43, 178,
    182–184, 186, 195, 196t
  in physical examination, 162
  pregnancy and, 143
  treatment of, 47–49
  in women, 140
  ZDV and, 35
Pneumonia, 13, 168, 185, 186
  bacterial, 154
  CMV, 44, 64
  interstitial, *see* Interstitial
    pneumonia
  Pneumocystis carinii, see
    Pneumocystis carinii
    pneumonia
Podophyllin, 127
POL gene, 24, 25, 38
Polymerase chain reaction
  (PCR), 180, 181, 182
Polyneuropathies, 162
Port-a-Cath catheters, 234
Postpartum transmission, 244
Postpartum treatment, 144
Posttest counseling, 25, 27,
  30–32
Poverty, 256
PPD test, *see* Purified protein
  derivative test
PPE, *see* Personal protective
  equipment; Pruritic
  papular eruption

Pregnancy, 29, 31, 137, 139,
  142–144, 146, *see also*
  Maternal transmission
Pretest counseling, 27–28, 29–30
Prevention, 243–258
  in health care workers, 244,
    247–252
  in individuals, 244–247
  in minority groups, 252–258
Primary brain lymphoma,
  58–60, 162
Primary infection treatment,
  35–38
Primary syphilis, 88, 89, 90, 91,
  95t, 141, 194
Prisoners, 51
Proctitis, 164
Progressive multifocal
  leukoencephalopathy, 54,
  93, 155, 162
Prostatitis, 164
Prostitutes, 245, 246, 263
Protease inhibitors, 25, 35, 38,
  see also specific types
Proteinuria, 107
Pruritic papular eruption
  (PPE), 131
Pseudomembranous colitis, 158
Psoriasis, 129–130
Psychiatric disorders, 264–266,
  see also specific types
Psychosocial aspects, 261–270
  care giver response to, 266–267,
    268–269
  evaluation of, 170–171
  management guidelines for,
    268–270
  nurses' assessment of, 223
  of pediatric HIV, 197–198, 263,
    264
  in women, 146, 264
Pulmonary disease, 168–170
Pulmonary Kaposi's sarcoma
  (KS), 44
Pulmonary support, 183, 184

Pulmonary system
    CMV and, 64
    examination of, 155, 162–163
Purified protein derivative
    (PPD) test, 52, 166
Pyrazinamide, 52, 53, 103t, 121,
    185
Pyridoxine, 52
Pyrimethamine, 54–55, 103t,
    108, 118

Quinolone, 52, 140

Race, *see* Minority groups;
    specific racial, ethnic groups
Radiation therapy, 60, 134
Rapid antigen testing, 186
Rapid plasma reagin (RPR),
    141, 166
Rashes, 158b, 186
Recombinant coagulation
    factors, 247
Rectal candidiasis, 154
Rectal examination, 164
Rectal placement of objects, 10
Renal dialysis, 78
Renal dysfunction, 103,
    106–108, 119–120
Renal failure, 183
Respiratory syncytial virus
    (RSV), 182, 185–186
Respiratory system,
    examination of, 154
Reticulocytosis, 186
Retin-A, 126
Retinitis, 168
    CMV, 64, 65, 160, 236
Retroviruses, 21–24, 35
Reverse transcriptase, 21, 22f,
    25, 38
Reverse transcriptase
    inhibitors, 35, 37
Rhinorrhea, 187
Ribavirin, 186
Ribonuclease H, 38

Rifabutin, 70, 71, 132
Rifampin, 52, 53, 103t, 120t, 121,
    185
Rigors, 156b
Ringworm, 128
Risk factors
    evaluation of, 153
    for hepatitis, 78
    for neutropenia, 108
    for pancreatitis, 106
    for peripheral neuropathy, 104
    for renal dysfunction, 107
RNA, 21, 25, 84
RNA probes, 52
RPR, *see* Rapid plasma reagin
RSV, *see* Respiratory syncytial
    virus

Safe sex, 29–30, 32, 205, 246,
    247, 262–263, 269
Salicylic acid ointment, 130
Saliva, 9, 243, 248
    CMV in, 64
Salmonella, 154, 170
Salmonellosis, 153, 158
San Francisco, 1
Scabies, 132–133, 160, 164
Sclerosing cholangitis, 120, 121
Seborrheic dermatitis, 129, 154, 160
Secondary syphilis, 88, 90, 141,
    194
    clinical manifestations of, 89
    diagnosis of, 92
    in physical examination, 160
    treatment of, 95t
Seizures, 41, 155
    CNS toxoplasmosis and, 53
    cryptococcal meningitis and, 56
    ddI and, 36
    primary brain lymphoma and,
        58
    syphilis and, 91
Semen, 9, 243–244
    CMV in, 64
Sensory neuropathies, 162

Septicemia, 234
Severe combined
    immunodeficiency, 15
Sexual transmission, 23, 243, 262
    of CMV, 64
    of condyloma, 126
    epidemiology of, 9
    of hepatitis, 78
    of pediatric HIV, 177, 180
    of syphilis, 87
SGOT, 120, 121, 166
SGPT, 120, 121, 166
Shigella, 154, 170
Shigellosis, 158
Shingles, 123, 124–125, *see also*
    Zoster
Side effects, *see* Adverse drug
    reactions
Sinusitis, 154
Skin, examination of, 154,
    160–161, *see also*
    Dermatologic
    manifestations
Smoking, 32
SMX, *see* Sulfamethoxazole
Snout reflex, 161
Social aspects, *see* Psychosocial
    aspects
Social workers, 4, 203–212
    evaluation by, 204–207
    interventions by, 207–211
Spermicides, 246
Spleen, 23
Splenomegaly, 70, 116, 118
Sponge, cervical, 145
Sputum analysis, 169, 184
Squamous cell carcinoma, 126,
    127
Sterilization, surgical, 145
Streptomycin, 52
Suicidal ideation, 31, 266
    nursing assessment of, 221–223
    social worker assessment of,
        205–206, 209–211
Sulfadiazine, 54–55, 103t, 107

Sulfa drugs, 120t
Sulfamethoxazole (SMX),
    143–144, *see also*
    Trimethoprim-
    sulfamethoxazole
Sulfonamides, 108
Support systems, 206, 207, 209,
    225–226
Suppressor T cells, 17
Surface antigens, 80, 81, 82, 251,
    252
Surface immunoglobulins, 16, 17
Sweat, 9
Symptomatic infections, 165t,
    166–170
Syndrome of inappropriate
    antidiuretic hormone
    secretion, 119–120
Syphilis, 43, 87–96, 155
    clinical manifestations of,
        87–88, 89–91
    congenital, 186–195
    diagnosis of, 91–95
    incubation period of, 88
    laboratory data on, 166, 167
    latent, *see* Latent syphilis
    medical history of, 153
    neuro-, *see* Neurosyphilis
    in physical examination, 164
    primary, *see* Primary syphilis
    secondary, *see* Secondary
        syphilis
    tertiary, 90, 140, 194
    treatment of, 95–96
    in women, 138, 141
Syphilitic arthritis, 90
Syphilitic hepatitis, 90
Systemic fungal infections,
    128–129
Systems review, 154–159

T cell leukemogenic
    retroviruses, 23, 24
T cells, 16, *see also specific types*
T3 (CD2) cells, 17

T4 (CD4) cells, 9, 13, 17–18, 19,
    23, 24, 32, 41, 161, *see also*
    Absolute T4 (CD4) cell
    count
  categories of, 151t
  ddC and, 37
  EPF and, 131
  hepatitis and, 83–84
  KS and, 133, 134
  MAC and, 71
  pancreatitis and, 106
  PCP and, 48
  pediatric HIV and, 178, 179t,
    196
  pediatric PCP and, 195
  peripheral neuropathies and,
    104
  PGL and, 43
  pregnancy and, 143, 144
  syphilis and, 92
  ZDV and, 35–36, 37
T4:T8 cell ratio, 43, 115, 167,
    178, 179t
T8 (CD8) cells, 17, 43, 115, 167,
    178, 179t
T4 lymphopenia, 178
Tabes dorsalis, 91
Tat inhibitors, 37–38
Tears, 9, 243
Tegretol, 125
Tertiary syphilis, 90, 141, 194
Texas, 11
Thrombocytopenia, 49, 118, 166
Thrush, *see* Oral candidiasis
Tinea, 127–128, 164
Tinea corporis, 128
Tinea cruris, 128
Tinea pedis, 127–128
Tinea versicolor, 160
TMP, *see* Trimethoprim
Tonsils, 23
Toxoplasma gondii, 18, 53, 167
Toxoplasmosis, 43, 93, 155
  CNS, 53–55, 162
  epidemiology of, 12

laboratory data on, 168
  in physical examination, 160,
    162
Transbronchial biopsies, 169
Transforming retroviruses, 22
Transmission, *see also*
    Prevention
  epidemiology of, 7–10
  modes of, 9–10, 171t, 243–244,
    see also specific modes
Transmission groups, 7–9
Traveler's diarrhea, 158
Treatment
  of ADC, 61
  of CMV, 65–66
  of CNS toxoplasmosis, 54–55
  of cryptococcal meningitis,
    57–58
  of *Cryptosporidium,* 68
  of esophageal candidiasis,
    66–67
  of hepatitis, 82–84
  of histoplasmosis, 50–51
  of *M. tuberculosis,* 52–53
  of MAC, 70–71
  of oral candidiasis, 66–67
  of PCP, 47–49
  of PGL, 43
  of primary brain lymphoma, 60
  of primary infection, 35–38
  of syphilis, 95–96
Treponemal assays, 94t, 95
Treponema pallidum, 87, 187
Trichomegaly, 132
Tricyclic antidepressants, 125
Trimethoprim-sulfamethoxazole
    (TMP-SMX), 47, 132, 169,
    195, 196t
  adverse reactions of, 48, 118,
    121, 183
Tuberculosis, 13, 43
  CNS toxoplasmosis confused
    with, 54
  immunology and, 18
  laboratory data on, 166, 169

medical history of, 153, 154
Mycobacterium, 51–53, 70, 166
pediatric HIV and, 182, 184–185
in physical examination, 160, 162
Tuberculosis meningitis, 155
Tuberculosis tests, 93
Tuskegee Syphilis Study, 255

Ultraviolet B radiation, 130–131
United States
  epidemiology in, 7, 8
  hepatitis in, 78, 81
  M. tuberculosis in, 51
Urine, 9, 243
  CMV in, 64
Urolagnia, 9

Vaccinations
  for HIV, 38
  in pediatric HIV cases, 197, 198t
Vaginal candidiasis, 138, 142–143, 154
Vaginal intercourse, 9, 246
Vaginal placement of objects, 10
Varicella zoster virus (VZV), 124–125, *see also specific diseases caused by*
VDRL, *see* Venereal Disease Research Laboratory
Venereal Disease Research Laboratory (VDRL), 92–95, 139, 141, 166, 187, 191, 193, 194
Verrucae vulgare, 126
Vinblastine, 134
Vincristine, 134
Viral cultures, 180, 182
Viral infections, 159, 170, *see also specific types*
  dental manifestations of, 214t
  dermatologic, 124–127
  immunology and, 16
Virazole, 186

Visual disturbances, 157b, *see also specific types*
Vitamin B$_{12}$, 104, 117
VZV, see Varicella zoster virus

Warts, 126–127, *see also* Condyloma
Weakness, 154
Weeping dermatitis, 248
Weight loss, 154, 156b
Western blot test, 113, 166
White blood cell count, 43, 57, 111
Whites, 11
Women, 2, 137–146
  diagnosis in, 138
  epidemiology of disease in, 8, 11, 137
  HIV testing in, 138
  intial work-up for, 139–140
  medical complications in, 140–144
  in minority groups, 252, 255, 257
  postpartum treatment of, 144
  psychosocial issues for, 146, 264

Xerosis, 131–132, 160

Zalcitabine (ddC), 36, 37, 38, 103t, 104, 105, 121
ZDV, *see* Zidovudine
Zidovudine (ZDV), 25, 167
  for ADC, 61
  adverse reactions of, 36, 103t, 108, 197
  for genital ulcers, 142
  for pediatric HIV, 180, 195–197
  for pediatric LIP, 184
  pregnancy and, 143, 144
  primary infection treated with, 35–36, 37, 38
  for psoriasis, 130
Zoster, 18, 153, 154, 160, *see also* Shingles
Zovirax, *see* Acyclovir

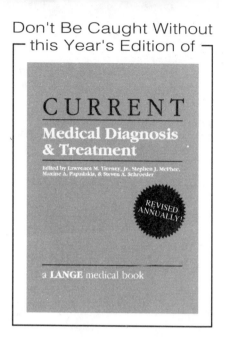